Fish oil and blood-vessel wall interactions

In order to respect the publication schedule, I did the papers modifications requested by the editor and proof corrections.
I hope authors will not mind too much and will excuse me if add mistakes appear in this text.
Thank you very much.

J. Daver, M.D., Ph. D
Science et Communication

Fish oil and blood-vessel wall interactions

Proceedings of the International Symposium held in Granada (Spain) February 23-25, 1990

Editors

P.M. Vanhoutte
Ph. Douste-Blazy

Pierre Fabre

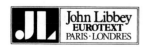
John Libbey
EUROTEXT
PARIS·LONDRES

British Library Cataloguing in Publication Data
Vanhoutte, P.M. (Paul M)
  Fish oil and blood-vessel wall interactions.
  1. Humans. Blood vessels. Drug therapy
  I. Title II. Douste-Blazy, Ph.
  616.13061

ISBN 0 86 196 294 X

Editions John Libbey Eurotext
6, rue Blanche, 92120 Montrouge, France.
Tél. : (1) 47.35.85.52 – Fax : (1) 46.57.10.09

John Libbey and Company Ltd
13, Smith Yard, Summerley Street, London SW18 4HR, England
Tél. : (81) 947.27.77

John Libbey CIC
Via L. Spallanzani, 11
00161 Rome, Italy
Tel. : (06) 862.289

Contents

Preface

The symposium on "fish oil and blood-vessel wall interaction" organised by the Pierre Fabre Laboratories and presided by P.M. Vanhoutte and Ph. Douste-Blazy has provided a general view of the influence of the endothelium in the regulation of circulatory and micro-circulatory phenomena, atherosclerosis and thrombosis. In particular, it emphasized that the role of endothelium derived relaxing factor (EDRF) appears to be fundamental.

In the context of these advances in our knowledge of regulatory mechanisms for the general circulatory system the highlighting of the important role of cellular elements represents undoubtedly the major breakthrough of recent years. In this respect two types of cells are particularly interesting : platelets because of their fundamental role in hemostasis, and as mediator vectors; and the endothelial cell, which are vitally important in both the local control of vascular tone and the prevention of thrombosis.

This international symposium was an opportunity not only to assess of recent advances in the fields of atherosclerosis, lipids, and blood vessels, but also to pinpoint certain pharmacological activities and the clinical interest of fish oils (Ω-3 fatty acid*) for the improvment of vascular protective mechanisms. The mechanisms underlying the beneficial effects of fish oils with a high Ω-3 fatty acid content are, complex and intricate and include :

- as far as lipids are concerned, a significant decrease in triglycerides and VLDL cholesterol, due in all probability to a reduction in the hepatic synthesis of lipoproteins and very low density proteins containing apolipoprotein B100;
- as far as the platelets are concerned, an inhibition to aggregation and decrease of thromboxane A2 synthesis, resulting in a possible preventive effect for thromboses;
- as far as the blood is concerned, a reduce viscosity and an increase deformability of red cells favoring the fluidity of the blood.

The endothelial cells of the arterial wall play an important physiological role. They synthesize various substances able to act as either vaso-dilators or as vaso-constrictors, and thus modify the reactivity of vascular smooth muscle. The functional importance of the underlying arterial endothelium

---

* Maxepa[®]

justifies measures taken to prevent its deterioration, notably by means of the use of Ω-3 polyunsaturated fatty acids. Indeed endothelial cells play a key role in vascular physiology and physiopathology. Functional anomalies generated in these cells by hypertension, arterial spasm, atherosclerosis or thrombosis govern complex changes in vascular equilibrium, on which it is sometimes difficults to act. It is therefore essential to strive to prevent these functional disturbances. It is likely that long term treatment by polyunsaturated Ω-3 fatty acids (fish oils) can prevent the functional deterioration of the endothelial cell by maintaining healthy physiological environmental conditions and by favoring the regeneration of these cells which inevitably decline with age.

P.M. Vanhoutte

Fish oil and blood-vessel wall interactions. Eds P.M. Vanhoutte, Ph. Douste-Blazy.
John Libbey Eurotext, Paris © 1991, pp 1-8.

1

Regulation of the cholesterol level in the plasma and mechanisms underlying hypercholesterolemia

Ph. Douste-Blazy*, G. Luc**

* *Atherosclerosis and Dislipidemia Risk Factor Prevention Unit,*
Cardiology Dept., Toulouse Regional Hospital Centre, Place Dr-Baylac
31059 Toulouse Cedex, France.
** *Lipoprotein and Atherosclerosis Research Dept. Pasteur Institute,*
1, rue du Pr-Calmette 59019 Lille Cedex, France.

Abstract

Cholesterol concentration depends essentially on the level of low-density lipoproteins (LPL). This in turn depends on genetic factors (LDL receptors, E phenotype apolipoprotein) and environmental factors (cholesterol, diet containing fatty acids). Hypercholesterolemia resulting from a high plasma level of LDL is one of the major risk factors in coronary great disease. A reduction of catabolism and/or and increase of LDL synthesis can be responsible for plasma abnormality. Among mechanisms which cause decreased catabolism, a deficiency in LDL receptors is the most well-known and corresponds most frequently to familial hypercholesterolemia. The presence of LDL anti-receptor anti-bodies is described; abnormalities in regulation of the number of LDL receptors are likely and could be characteristic of most cases of hypercholesterolemia; these anomalies are probably aggravated by a high lipid diet A B100 apolipoprotein mutation involving a decrease of LDL binding to its receptors is shown to be a cause of hypercholesterolemia. Cholesterol is carried by all types of lipoprotein particles (cf. Cholesterol : where does it come from ? How does it circulate ? Where does it go ?) However about 70 % of plasma cholesterol is carried by low density lipoproteins (LDLs) in normal human plasma while the proportion is 20 to 30 % for that carried by high density lipoproteins (HDLs). This 20 % to 30 % is not subject to major quantitative variations although the biological variations may be considerable. Plasma cholesterol concentration therefore depends primarily on that of the LDLs.

Ph. Douste-Blazy, G. Luc

Cholesterolemia regulation

LDL concentration depends on genetic and environmental factors which influence the catabolism or the synthesis of these particles. The importance of the role of LDL regulators in LDL catabolism has been mentioned, as has the fact that a modification in the number of LDL receptors leads to variable cholesterolemia. Another genetic factor is the apo E phenotype. Apo E is a protein consisting of 299 amino-acids on the surface of lipoproteins rich in triglycerides and HDLs. Different forms of apo E have been recognised, these being the consequence of genetic variations. There are 3 common forms of Apo E : E2, E3 and E4 leading to the presence in the population of 6 different phenotypes, the most common of these being E3/3. Several groups have noted that, in normo-lipidic subjects, the LDL level is higher in those with an E4/4 or an E4/3 phenotype (which contains the allele E4) than in those with an E3/3 phenotype, (or an E2/2 phenotype where the LDL is lower still). These differences are connected to the presence of a greater number of hepatic LDL receptors in E2/2 phenotype subjects than in those with an E3/3 phenotype, (or E4/4 where the number of LDL receptors is lower still). The resulting consequence is a variable LDL catabolism depending on the apo E phenotype. A recent study carried out among octogenarian subjects has shown an almost total absence of E4/4 and E4/3 phenotypes, suggesting that phenotype E4 has a considerable influence on longevity, in all probability through the presence of a more rapid atherogenesis connected to a higher level of LDL due to apo E phenotype.

High cholesterol food increases the LDL plasma concentration. With this type of diet the greater quantity of cholesterol absorbed is carried by the chylomicrons which are retained by the liver after lypolysis. Cholesterol thus delivered to the liver is used in the synthesis of liver secreted lipoproteins (VLDLs) which are high in cholesterol and converted into LDLs. It has moreover been shown that, with this type of diet, the activity of HMG Co Reductase (an intercellular enzyme with a role in cholesterol synthesis) is decreased. This decrease has a parallel in the decreased activity of the LDL receptors. The increased cholesterol brought to the hepatocytes by the remnants of the chylomicrons diminishes LDL receptor activity through negative retroactive control; LDL catabolism is therefore decelerated. The consequence is an increased concentration of plasma LDL. It must however be born in mind that the modification of plasma cholesterol is highly from one

2

subject to another. The cause probably lies in a variable regulation of the activity of LDL receptors in different subjects.

It is also well known that a diet rich in saturated fatty acids increases LDL levels and hence plasma cholesterol concentration, while a diet rich in poly-unsaturated fatty acids causes a decrease of LDLs and a slight drop in HDLs. Mono-unsaturated fatty acids seem not to have the disadvantage of reducing the HDL level, while at the same time maintaining an LDL concentration similar to that of a diet rich in poly-unsaturated fatty acids [2].

Mechanisms of hypercholesterolemia

Pathological hypercholesterolemia is always the result of an increase in the plasma concentration of low density lipoproteins (LDLs). The particles are atherogenous and there is a connection between LDL cholesterol concentration and coronary mortality. In this context, hypercholesterolemia can be defined as an LDL cholesterol level above 3.36 mmol/l (1.30 g/l). This article will not deal with hypercholesterolemia brought on by an increase in HDLs (high density lipoproteins) which can cause an increase in plasma cholesterol even if LDL cholesterol is normal. Subjects exhibiting this anomaly (hyper-alphalipoproteinemia) whose condition could be described as a false hyper-cholesterolemia, have a lengthy survival rate. Advances in our knowledge of the physiopathology of hypercholesterolemia have been based on new biological techniques (monoclonal antibodies, molecular biology) It has been shown, with the aid of these techniques, that the mechanisms leading to hypercholesterolemia are varied. Hypercholesterolemia could thus be the result of an increase in the synthesis, or a decelaration in the catabolism of LDLs.

Hypercholesterolemia by decreased LDL Catabolism

Hypercholesterolemia due to an LDL receptor deficiency

This mechanism corresponds primarily to familial hypercholesterolemia. Familial hypercholesterolemia is a frequent monogenic autosomal dominant illness (1/500 births). Its clinical characteristics are extra-vascular deposits, tendinous xanthomas (Achilles tendons, finger extensor tendons) as well as xanthelasma, tuberous xanthomas and in some serious cases (homozygous) flat cutaneous xanthomas. The primary cause of the significant increase in

LDLs found in this condition is a decrease is the number of LDL receptors. This deficiency is apparent both in the case of cultured fibroblasts taken from such patients, and hepatic membranes obtained after surgical biopsy [3, 4]. Two types exist depending on whether the condition is heterozygous or homozygous. The homozygous condition is characterised by a functional impairment of the LDL receptors coded by the chromosomes (chromosomes 19) originating in the two parents. Specific LDL binding on to the cells of these patients is in this case less than 30 % of normal binding (< 5 % : receptor negative, between 5 and 30 % : receptor defective). Sometimes the LDL binding to their receptor is normal but the LDL-receptor complex is not internalised in the cell (internalisation defect). Receptor studies have shown that several different mutations giving rise to the same phenotypical disturbances, can be detected in homozygous subjects.

We are currently aware or 4 categories :

1 – no precursory synthesis;

2 – LDL anomaly in LDL receptor transmission from endoplasmatic reticulum to the Golgi mechanism;

3 – LDL to receptor binding anomaly;

4 – LDL internalisation defect.

Familial studies have revealed that some homozygotes (55 %) are in fact double heterozygotes (with a different anomaly originating in each of two hypercholesterolemic parents, the remaining 45 % being true homozygotes (the two chromosomes possessing the same anomaly).

The reduction in the number of receptors leads to lengthier LDL plasma residence (LDL half life being 5.2 days in homozygotes, 3.75 days in heterozygotes, and 2.1 days in normal subjects) [5]. This increase leads to a rise in LDL levels. But there is also an increase in LDL synthesis, negligeable or non-existant in heterozygous subjects, but significant in homozygotes. This synthesis could be derived directly from the liver, or could be the consequence of increased VLDL catabolism. The mechanism of LDL overproduction has been to a certain extent clarified by studies on Watanabe heritable hyperlipidemic (WHHL) mutant rabbits whose LDL receptor level is less than 5 %. This animal model of familial hypercholesterolemia shows vascular and extra-vascular deposits similar to those found in the human patient.These rabbits are without hepatic IDL (lipoproteins produced by VLDL catabolism) retention. These IDL are almost entirely transformed into LDL whereas in the normal rabbit 90 % are retained by the liver [4]. In people, while this mechanism is instrumental, it does not entirely explain LDL over production, almost all of the IDLs being converted into LDL in the normal subject.

The LDL level in a homozygous hypercholesterolemic subject being stable and LDL production being two or three times that of a normal subject, LDL catabolism in hypercholesterolemic subjects is this high but takes place through processes in which the receptors are not involved. However, in the WHHL rabbit, the distribution per organ of LDL catabolism is similar to that of the normal rabbit (65 % by the liver). Thus the mechanisms which are quantitatively simimar but biologically different have different consequences on the LDL. In the human homozygous subject, the specific LDL bonding to the hepatic membranes is only reduced by 50 % and the biological characteristics of the LDL receptors seem to be partially different from those of the usual fibroblast description. Hepatic regulation would thus seem to be different from that of peripheral tissues. However the degradation of the hepatic receptors does play a significant part in LDL metabolism in the homozygous hypercholesterolemic subject since a child subject of a double liver-heart transplant subsequently experienced considerable improvement in its LDL catabolism.

The presence of LDL anti-receptor antibodies

While seeking the cause of major hypercholesterolemia (6-9 g/l) in a patient with no family background of disease, or of atherosclerosis, the type "IgA" LDL anti-receptor antibodies were discovered. This antibody, when incubated with normal fibroblasts inhibits LDL bonding; it has been shown that this paraprotein interacts directly with the LDL receptor [7].

Anomaly connected to receptor dysregulation

In addition to LDL receptor structural anomalies, there are also anomalies of receptor expression on the surface of the cells. A child has been reported with a clinical and biological phenotype corresponding to homozygous familial hypercholesterolemia; however, this phenotype corresponded to normal receptor expression on cultured cells except that it was for an abnormally high intracellular cholesterol requirement [8]. The *in vivo* study of LDL catabolism has shown a deceleration similar to that of homozygous familial hypercholesterolemia. This case, although caricatural, may well appear in a less noticeable form in other cases of moderate hypercholesterolemia.

The interaction between a slight anomaly in the LDL receptor gene and environmental factors such as diet could lead to hypercholesterolemia. In the human subject an increase in the cholesterol content of the diet involves a variable rise in cholesterol level. The plasma LDL cholesterol increase is negatively correlated to the activity of monocyte reductase HMG CoA (reflecting the LDL receptor bonding) [9]. The cholesterol increase induced by a high cholesterol diet is more significant in subjects affected by familial hypercholesterolemia, a disease in which there is already an LDL receptor anomaly. Regulation of the number of LDL receptors therefore seems to be of some importance in dietary response and a minimum of dysregulation could be a cause of hypercholesterolemia.

Gene segments responsible for LDL receptor expression and HMG Co reductase are now known and mutation here, although this has not yet been demonstrated, could be responsible for hypercholesterolemia.

Anomaly due to an abnormal apolipoprotein

LDLs are catabolised through specific bonding of the protein present on their surface, apo B100, to their receptor. If there is a mutation here the affinity of the LDLs for their receptors can be altered. The LDLs would then be decomposed more slowly thus inducing hypercholesterolemia.

Thus, we have seen that certain subjects with moderate hypercholesterolemia experience LDL decomposition more slowly than in normo-lipidemic subjects when the two types of LDL (normal and hypercholesterolemia) are injected simultaneously into either normo-lipidemic, difference is therefore not due to the LDL receptor since a pharmacological increase in the number of LDL receptors (treatment with a HMG CoA reductase called lovastatine) does not modify the results.

In a family whose propositus showed these conditions, an anomaly of the LDL apo-B100 (modification of an amino-acid due to the mutation of the gene base) is responsible, since the LDL affinity of these subjects is less than for the LDL of normal subjects, even though the physical and chemical characteristics of his LDLs were normal [12].

Hypercholesterolemia through increased LDL synthesis

Some cases of hypercholesterolemia do not appear to be due to an LDL catabolism defect, but to inordinate LDL synthesis which results in a new synthesis/catabolism balance, but at the cost of hypercholesterolemia. The plasma cholesterol and LDL levels are very variable, sometimes extremely high (5 g/l in one child, a personal case) although they are generally moderate (2.5 to 3 g/l) This latter case seems often to correspond to combined familial hyperlipidemia in its IIa phenotype form. This hyperlipidemia described by Goldstein in 1973 and based on genetic investigations among survivors of myocardial infarctus is probably the most frequent genetically transmitted atherogenous hyperlipidemia [13].

It is characterised by the presence in the same family of variable lipoprotein phenotypes of the types IIa, IIb, IV and exceptionally V. Genetic investigation will therefore uncover in one member affected by hyperlipidemia either hypercholesterolemia through LDL increase (type IIa) or isolated hyper-triglyceridemia through increased VLDL (type IV), or again a simultaneous increase in cholesterol and triglycerides (type IIb). The phenotype can moreover vary in the same subject in the course of time and the frequency of these phenotypes in the same family is also variable. The lipid increase appears in adulthood and the mode of transmission is not yet clearly established – it may be autosomal dominant, or polygenic [14].

Increase in apo-B100 production can be caused by different anomalies. An excessive synthesis of apo-B100 can be the direct consequence of disregulation or can be due to another lipidic anomaly. Thus a protein called "Acylating Stimulating Protein" (ASP) which stimulates the synthesis of triglycerides in the adipose cells is inversely correlated to the LDL apo-B concentration. Hence a reduction in the build-up of fatty acid reserves in the adipose tissue (in the form of triglycerides) increases the volume of fatty acids reaching the liver which consequently proceeds to an excessive synthesis of triglycerides and VLDL [15].

Conclusion

A better knowledge of the physiopathology of hypercholesterolemia on the one hand, and of the mechanism of different hypolipodemiants on the other hand, permits more suitable treatment of these diseases which are responsible for atheroma, particularly of the coronary, one of the major public health problems of the industrialised world.

References

1. Sing CF, Davignon J. Role of the apolipoprotein E polymorphism in determining normal lipid and lipoprotein variation. Am J Hum Gen 1985; 37 : 268-285.

2. Grundy SM, Vega GL. Plasma cholesterol responsiveness to saturated fatty acids. Am J Clin Nutr 1988; 47 : 822-824.

3. Goldstein JL, Brown MS. Binding and degradation of low density lipoproteins by cultured human fibroblasts : comparison of cells from a normal subject and from a patient with homozygous hypercholesterolemia. J Biol Chem 1974; 249 : 5153-5182.

4. Hoeg JM, Demosky SJ, Shaeffer EJ. Characterization of hepatic low density lipoprotein binding and cholesterol metabolism in normal and homozygous familial hypercholesterolemic subjects. J. Clin Invest 1984; 73 : 429-436.

5. Packard CJ, Third JLHC, Shepherd J *et al.* Low density lipoprotein metabolism in a family of familial hypercholesterolemic patients. Metabolism 1976; 25 : 995-1006.

6. Goldstein JL, Kita T, Brown MS. Defective lipoprotein receptors and atherosclerosis. N Engl J Med 1983; 309 : 288-296.

7. Corsini A, Roma P, Sommariva D *et al.* Autoantibodies to the low density lipoprotein receptor in a subject affected by severe hypercholesterolemia. J Clin Invest 1986; 78 : 940-946.

8. De Gennes JL, Luc G, Benhamamouch S *et al.* Abnormal expression of low-density lipoprotein receptors in a Lebanese family : defective expression *in vivo* and *in vitro* of low density lipoprotein receptors in a child presenting hypercholesterolemia. Arteriosclerosis (submitted).

9. Mistry P, Miller NE, Laker M. Individual variation in the effects od dietary cholesterol on plasma lipoproteins and cellular cholesterol homeastasis in man. J Clin Invest 1981; 67 : 493-502.

10. Brown MS. 8th International Symposium on Atherosclerosis, Roma 1988.

11. Vega Gl, Grundy SM. *In vivo* evidence for reduced binding of low density lipoproteins to receptors as a cause of primary hypercholesterolemia. J Clin Invest 1986; 78 : 1410-1414.

12. Innerarity TL, Weisgraber KH, Arnold KS *et al.* Familial defective apolioprotein B100 : low density lipoproteins with abnormal receptor binding. Proc Natl Acad Sci USA 1987; 84 : 6919-6923.

13. Goldstein JL, Schrott HG, Hazzard WR *et al.* Hyperlipidemia in coronary heart disease II. Genetic analysis op lipid levels in 176 families and delineation of a new disorder, combined hyperlipidemia. J Clin Invest 1973; 52 : 1544-1568.

14. Grundy SM, Chait A, Brunzell JD. Familial combined hyperlipidemia; Workshop. Arteriosclerosis 1987; 7 : 203-207.

15. Sniderman AD. Hyper apo-B. 8th International Symposium on Atherosclerosis. Workshop Sessions, Roma 1988, p. 44.

Fish oil and blood-vessel wall interactions. Eds P.M. Vanhoutte, Ph. Douste-Blazy.
John Libbey Eurotext, Paris © 1991, pp. 9-16.

2

Platelets and arterial thrombosis

M. Dechavanne

*Hemobiology laboratory INSERM U331, Lyon Pasteur Institute,
A.-Carrel Medical Faculty, rue, Guillaume-Paradin, 69372 Lyon Cedex 08.*

Abstract

The results of anatomical, pathological, biological and therapeutic studies tend to support the hypothesis that platelets play a role in the formation of arterial thrombosis. The platelet thrombus is constantly present in contact with the damaged vascular wall. On the occasion of acute thrombotic episodes an increase in platelet activation by indicators such as β-thromboglobulin, or thromboxane B_2 can be seen. Lastly, the use of acetyl-salicylic acid decreases thrombosis mortality and relapse when treatment is undertaken during the acute phase of myocardial infarction, unstable angine, or subsequent to myocardial infarction. Platelets favorise the development of atherosclerosis and are active in several ways in the formation of arterial thrombosis : they adhere to damaged vessels, then become active, and aggregate. At the same time, they facilitate the generation of thrombine which stabilises the platelet thrombus and forms fibrin. Lastly the platelet thrombus has greater resistance to plasmin lysis than a fibrin thrombus.

The thrombus created after damage to a vessel is partly composed of platelets. A significant decrease in their number in the blood composition or a major deficiency in one of their functions is accompanied by hemorrhages in particular at the microvascular level. These clinical observations constitute an essential proof of the role of platelets in hemostasis : they contribute to vessel maintenance and close vascular breaches. Are they a causal factor in arterial thrombosis ? The reply is not a simple one. Experimental and *in vitro* studies have given us a better insight into the mechanisms of thrombosis; they indicate that platelets are active in arterial thrombosis and in atherosclerosis. In humans however we have no precise knowledge of the significance of platelets in the development of these two pathologies, which are both multi-factorial in nature.

Platelets favorise arterial thrombosis in man

This statement is based on the results of anatomical/pathological, biological and therapeutic studies.

Anatomical/pathological studies have shown the presence of platelets in the arterial thrombus for several years : their presence is constant but their activity varies from one thrombus to another. When the shearing forces exercised on the vessel by blood flow are weak the thrombus which is created consists essentially of fibrin enclosing the red corpuscles. When on the other hand these forces are strong, which is the case with atheromatous lesions, that part of the thrombus which adheres to the damaged vessel contains a very high proportion of platelets [1]. This suggests that the platelets could, after adhering to vascular lesions, become then active and aggregate.

Biological studies have highlighted platelet activation during arterial thrombosis. Thus during the acute stage of myocardial infarction, or in unstable angina, there is very often an increase in the plasma of substances such as beta thromboglobulin, secreted by the platelets under stimulus. In the same way the urinary metabolites of B_2 thromboxane are increased [3,4]. These are particularly indicative of the *in vivo* synthesis of A_2 thromboxane by the platelets; their level in fact decreases after the moderate administration of acetylsalicylic acid which inhibits the synthesis of A_2 thromboxane by the platelets [5]. The biological indicators of platelet activation are also increased in those clinical situations which favorise arterial thrombosis such as insulin dependent diabetes [6], stress [7] and tobacco use [8]. It is sometimes possible to reveal abnormal platelet attachment to an atheromatous artery be means of indium 111 marking [9]. On the other hand in venous thrombosis platelet activation is moderate and is always accompanied by coagulation [10].

Caution is necessary in the interpretation of these biological results. In fact all of these techniques are subject to artefacts : in particular the beta thromboglobulin plasma level depends on the quality of the blood sample and on the kidney's capacity to eliminate it [2]. Moreover the urinary levels of B_2 thromboxane metabolites (2, 3-dinor-thromboxane B_2 and 11 dehydrothromboxane B_2) vary from day to day by an average of 15 % in the same subject [11].

Again, the indium 111 marking of platelets requires manipulation which may deteriorate the platelets and modify their *in vivo* functions.

There have been numerous *therapeutic* trials using platelet anti-aggregants. It has been possible in three pathologies to highlight the efficacy of acetyl-salicylic acid on relapsed arterial thrombosis, and on vascular mortality. Subsequent to myocardial infarction, a simultaneous analysis covering the seven leading controled studies [12,13] has shown that after 1 year vascular morta-lity was reduced by 9 % in the groups treated with acetylsalicylic acid, compared to the placebo groups. Myocardial infarction relapse was decreased by 25 % : it stood at 5.6 % in the treated groups compared to 7.5 % in the placebo groups. The relapse of vascular accidents, whatever their type was, decreased by 20 % : the frequency of these accidents was 14.6 % in the treated groups *compared to* 17.6 % for the placebo groups. During the acute phase of myocardial infarctus, the ISIS-II study [14], involving more than 17 000 patients, showed that, after 5 weeks of treatment, mortality was re-duced by 23 % in the group receiving acetylsalicylic acid compared to the placebo group : it stood at 10.7 % in the treated group compared to 13.2 % in the placebo group. The effect was more noticeable still when acetylsali-cylic acid was accompanied by streptokinase; the decrease in mortality was then 42 % : 8 % of deaths in the group treated with streptokinase plus by acetylsalicylic acid. Streptokinase alone decreased mortality by only 28 %. In all groups treated with acetylsalicylic acid myocardial infarction relapse was decreased by half. In the case of unstable angina, three controled studies [15, 16, 17] have shown that vascular mortality and myocardial infarction relapse on the sixth day, and again at the 26th month were decreased in the group treated with acetylsalicylic [12,13]. Although, in the low doses used for most of these tests, this acid affects platelets by inhibiting the synthesis of A_2 thromboxane, its beneficial effect cannot be categorically attributed to its anti-platelet function.

Thus the results of anatomical/pathological, biological and therapeutic studies tend to coincide and to support the hypothesis of an active role played by the platelets in the development of arterial thrombosis.

Mechanism underlying the role of the platelets

Platelets are active in the development of the arterial thrombus and of atherosclerosis at several stages.

In humans they do not seem to be involved in the initial genesis of atherosclerosis. On the other hand they play a primordial role in the development of the atheromatous lesion. When the atheromous plaque becomes ulcerous this is generally followed by two major events : the creation of a thrombus in the region of the lesion and a hematoma of the wall. The most common outcome is for the situation to become chronic with stabilisation of the thrombus which becomes covered with endothelial cells and a deterioration of the haematoma. During these processes, the platelets release their lipidic components and their growth factors including platelet derived growth factor (PDGF). The macrophages accumulate lipids and become spumous. The smooth muscle cells in the aera are subjected to migration and proliferation due to the action of PDGF. Thus the atherosclerosis plaque gets bigger; it can become ulcerous again re-starting the same cycle. At a given moment in time it becomes large enough to decrease blood flow and set off clinical symptoms. These anatomical pathological observations have been confirmed by direct arterial investigation using angioscopy [18]. They show the close link between atherosclerosis and arterial thrombosis.

As soon as the endothelial cells are damaged the platelets adhere to the different components of the sub-endothelium. A fine layer of platelets is formed, without aggregation in a healthy vessel. On the other hand in the presence of atheromatous lesions, or if there is repeated disendothelialisation, the platelets adhere and become active; they secrete their dense and alpha granules and proceed to aggregate. Platelet adhesion is only partly understood. It is favorised by the number of circulating red blood cells and their capacity for deformation together with the shearing forces; these factors tend to project the platelets on to the sub-endothelium. In the adhesion process, the von Willebrand factor comes into play, a factor synthesised by the endothelial cells and the megacaryocytes. It is present in the plasma and platelets where it is stored in the alpha granules; it is secreted by the activated platelets. It allows the platelets to adhere to collagen and to the heparinoid substances of the sub-endothelium. The platelets possess two types of receptors for von Willebrand factor : Ib glycoprotein and the IIb-IIIa complex or αIIb-β_3 integrin. Other platelet receptors could bind to other structures of the sub-endothelium : platelet αv β_3 integrin to vitronectin, $\alpha\gamma\beta_3$ integrin to thrombospondin, α_5 β_1 integrin to fibronectin, α_6 β_1 integrin to laminin, and both α_2 β_1 integrin and IIIb glycoprotein to collagen (*Figure 1*).

Platelet activation favorises thrombus formation. In fact it leads to the secretion of platelet alpha and dense granules. These contain several substances including ADP and serotonin which prompt the aggregation of circulating platelets; in the same way activated platelets synthesise A_2 thromboxane which spreads out of the cell, activating circulating platelets and contracting the vessels. Lastly activation is characterized by a change in integrin con-

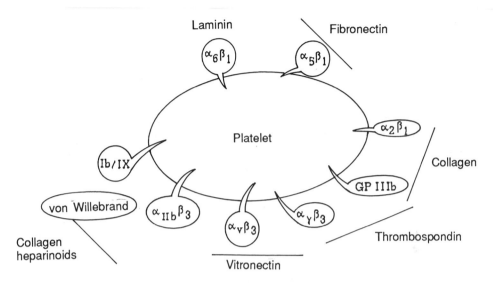

Figure 1. Structures implied in platelet adhesion to the sub-endothelium RGD peptids are specific of cyto-adhesins platelet receptors (fibronectin, thrombospondin, vitronectin, von Willebrand, etc.) They inhibit platelet adhesion.

formation; it becomes able to set the fibrinogen which cements the activated platelets together to make an aggregate. Ticlopidin inhibits platelet aggregation by adhering to this integrin and opposing its interaction with fibrinogen. Another membrane change is significant: the "flip-flop" phenomenon. This takes the form of a backfold of part of the membrane; its gives internal phospholipids such as phosphatidyl serine (to which plasma coagulation factors adhere) access to the outside surface. On contact with such a membrane these factors are activated; they create thrombin which, adhering to the platelet membrane, is no longer inhibited by antithrombin III.

The agonistic agents responsible for this platelet activation have not been identified. On the other hand, both the biochemical mechanisms which lead to granule secretion of dense and alpha, and synthetis of thromboxane A_2 are partly known. Agonists cause a structural modification of the membrane G proteins by adhering to its receptor : this is known as transduction *(Figure 2)*.

These G proteins regulate several enzymatic systems. G_p activates C phospholipase and Gi inhibits adenylate cyclase; activated C phospholipase deteriorates the membrane polyphosphoinositides (P1P2) to create diacyl-glycerol and inositol 1, 4, 5 triphosphate (IP3). Adenylate cyclase inhibition decreases the intra-cellular level of cyclic AMP. This decrease, to-

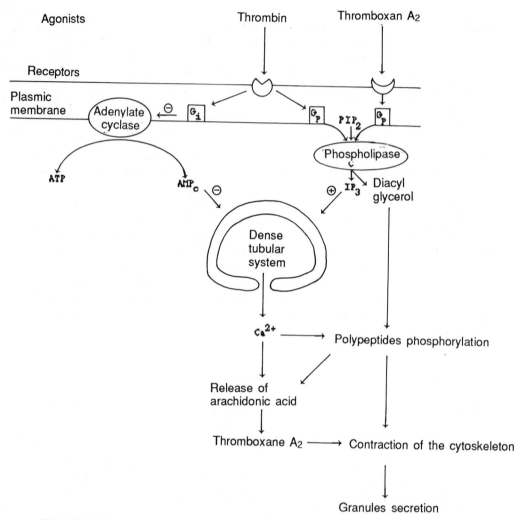

Figure 2. Main stages of platelet activation.

gether with an increase in IP3 level, cause mobilisation of the calcium of the dense tubular system which is a calcium storage organ. The accumulation of calcium in the cytoplasm and the presence of diacyl-glycerol activate the kinase protein, responsible for the phosphorylation of several polypeptides; this causes contraction of the cytoskeleton proteins and the secretion of platelets granules. It also triggers phospholipase A_2 activation with, as a consequence, the release of arachidonic acid which is transformed into thromboxane A_2 [19].

Lastly, platelets have an anti-thrombolytic activity. The *in vitro* lysis of a platelet enriched thrombus is incomplete compared with a fibrin thrombus. In the dog where we know how to create a fibrin-rich or platelet-rich thrombus according to the stimulation given, the perfusion with tissue plasminogenous activator (t-PA) at a 1mg/kg dose for 30 minutes breaks down the platelet-rich thrombus less often than the fibrin-rich one [20]. This effect could be linked to the secretion by the platelets of a t-PA inhibitor, PAI-1 [21]; it could also depend on the release of factor XIII by the platelets; this factor renders fibrin resistant to the action of plasmin [22].

Thus our knowledge of the role of platelets in arterial thrombosis is improving. Clinical applications of this knowledge should soon be forthcoming. The use of monoclonal antibodies, specific to platelet activation antigens, (GMP-140; $\alpha_2\beta_1$...) should allow the detection of activated *(ex vivo* and *in vivo)* platelets in damaged vessels. As far as therapy is concerned acetylsalicylic and ticlopidin remain the basic anti-aggregants for chronic treatment. However a new generation of molecules is making its appearance, with, particularly the RGD peptides, specific to cyto-adhesine platelet receptors, proteins which play a role in platelet adhesion *(Figure 1)* and fibrogenous platelet aggregation. Experimentally these peptides prevent re-occlusion after thrombolysis.

References

1. Freiman DG. The structure of thrombi. *In Hemostasis and thrombosis.* Colman RW, Hirsh J, Marder VS, Salzman EW (Eds) Philadelphia. JB Lippincott 1987; pp. 1123-1135.

2. Kaplan KL, Owen J. Plasma levels of β-thromboglobulin and platelet factor 4 as indices of platelet activation *in vivo.* Blood 1981; 57 : 199-202.

3. Fitzgerald DJ, Roy L, Catela F *et al*. Platelet activation in unstable coronary artery disease. New Engl J Med 1986; 315 : 983-989.

4. Henrikson P, Wennmalm A, Edhag O *et al. In vivo* production of prostacyclin and thromboxane in patients with acute myocardial infarction. Br Heart J 1986; 55 : 543-548.

5. Reilly IAG, Fitzgerald GA. Inhibition of thromboxane formation *in vivo* and *ex vivo* : implications for thepary with platelet inhibitory drugs. Blood 1987; 69 : 180-186.

6. Alessandrini P, McRae J, Feman S *et al*. Thromboxane biosynthesis and platelet function in type I diabetes mellitus. N Engl J Med 1988; 319 : 208-212.

7. Levine SP, Towell BL, Suarez AM *et al*. Platelet activation and secretion associated with emotional stress. Circulation 1985; 71 : 1129-1134.

8. Nowak J, Murray JJ, Oates JA *et al*. Biochemical evidence of a chronic abnormality in platelet and vascular function in healthy individuals who smoke cigarettes. Circulation 1987; 76 : 6-14.

9. Drouet LO, Mundler O, Fauchet M. Intérêt des plaquettes marquées à l'indium en pathologie thrombotique. Sang Thrombose Vaisseaux 1989; 1 : 77-88.

10. Harker LA, Slichter SJ. Platelet and fibrinogen consumption in man N Engl J Med 1972; 287 : 999-1005.

11. Catella F, Fitzgerald GA. Paired analysis of urinary thromboxane B_2 metabolites in humans. Thromb Res 1987; 47 : 647-656.

12. Antiplatelet trialist's collaboration. Secondary prevention of vascular disease by prolonged antiplatelet treatment. Br Med J 1988; 296 : 320-331.

13. Castaigne A, Duval-Moulin AM, Dutoit C. Antiagrégants plaquettaires et pathologie coronaire. Rev Prat 1989; 39 : 2228-2232.

14. ISIS-II. Collaborative group : Randomized trial of intravenous streptokinase, oral aspirin, both or neither among 17187 cases of suspected acute myocardial infarction. Lancet 1988; ii : 349-360.

15. Lewis HD, Davis JW, Archibald DG *et al.* Protective effects of aspirin against acute myocardial infarction and death in men with unstable angina. Results of a Veterans Administration cooperative study. N Engl J Med 1983; 309 : 396-403.

16. Cairns JA, Gent M, Singer J *et al.* Aspirin, sulfinpyrazone or both in unstable angina. Results of a Canadian multicenter trial. N Engl J Med 1985; 313 : 1369-1375.

17. Theroux P, Ouimet MP, McCans J *et al.* Aspirin, heparin, or both to treat acute unstable angina. N Engl J Med 1988; 319 : 1105-1111.

18. Forrester JS, Litvack F, Grundfest W *et al.* A perspective of coronary disease seen through the arteries of living man. Circulation 1987; 75 : 505-513.

19. Kroll MH, Schaffer AI. Biochemical mechanisms of platelet activation. Blood 1989; 74 : 1181-1195.

20. Haskel EJ, Adams SP, Feigen LP *et al.* Prevention of reoccluding platelet-rich thrombi in canine femoral arteries with a novel peptide antagonist of platelet glucoprotein IIb-IIIa receptors. Circulation 1989; 80 : 1775-1782.

21. Erickson LA, Ginsberg MH, Loskutoff DH. Detection and partial characterization of an inhibitor of plasminogen activator in human platelets. J Clin Invest 1984; 74 : 1465-1472.

22. Francis CW, Marder VJ. Increased resistance to plasmic degradation of fibrin with highly crosslinked α-polymer chains formed at high factor XIII concentrations. Blood 1985; 71 : 1361-1365.

Fish oil and blood-vessel wall interactions. Eds P.M. Vanhoutte, Ph. Douste-Blazy.
John Libbey Eurotext, Paris © 1991, pp. 17-36.

3

Microcirculation and microrheology

M.R. Boisseau

INSERM U8, Université de Bordeaux II, 33604 Pessac, France.

Introduction

Over the past decade, increasing attention has been paid to the role of the microcirculation in the pathophysiology of a number of conditions. A microcirculation has been identified anatomically in all major organs, and its physiological role has been investigated in various animal or experimental models. Despite the paucity of studies in humans, a considerable body of knowledge has now been accumulated which has formed the subject of numerous publications and reviews of which those of Tsuchiya [77], Messmer [48], Larcan [39], Mortillaro [50], Manabe [44], Wiedeman *et al.* [85] deserve mention. Over the same period, fundamental studies on blood flow in microvessels have been carried out, especially with respect to the movement of blood cells. This has given rise to the concept of microrheology. Even more recently, the role played by endothelial cells in microrheology via cell-cell interactions has become apparent.

A number of lines of evidence point to an intimate link between microrheological phenomena and the microcirculation. Although the microcirculation is under neuro-hormonal regulation and vasomotor control, both passive and active rheological processes occur essentially in the microcirculation, as they only become significant in vessels subjected to low propulsive forces. Such processes tend to be amplified under various pathological conditions. Considerable impairment of the microcirculation may occur in vascular disease, for example, and rheological disorders need to be taken into account when evaluating the patient's condition [9]. In fact, treatment strategies aimed specifically at disorders of blood cell rheology are under development.

This chapter will outline first the histological, physiological and pathophysiological aspects of the microvessels.

The microcirculation

Microvessels

Microvessels can be considered to include all vessels with a diameter or 100 µm or less. These vessels constitute the true capillary bed, the principle site of exchanges between blood and tissues. In fact, there is no clear-cut distinction between the systemic and the microcirculation, but vessels whose diameters are of a similar order of magnitude to the those of blood cells are subjected to different hemodynamic influences, and are much more sensitive to rheological factors. They constitute a considerable reservoir of blood especially on the venous side. On the arterial side, they represent a principle source of peripheral resistance which is regulated by the sympathetic branch of the autonomic nervous system.

The microvessels encompass a large surface area, and in man, the endothelial cells lining these vessels have been estimated to weigh 3 kg. The importance of the endothelial organ which is in constant contact with blood is highlighted by recently identified actions of this tissue on both blood and muscle cells in vessels walls.

Microcirculation as an entity

There are considerable differences in the functional arrangements of microvessels, especially in parenchymatous organs (see review by Wiedeman *et al.* [85]). A common functional unit can, however, be identified, typified by the microcirculation in muscles, which represents the largest area of microvessels in the organism. In France, the notion of the microcirculation unit has been extensively studied by Merlen (1912-1986).

Table I shows the constitution of the microcirculation unit in the vascular tree. It consists of five principle vessel types : arterioles (100 to 40 µ) surrounded by richly innervated smooth muscle cells : pre-capillary arterioles

Table 1. Position of microvessels in the circulatory system. *Diameter* : cm for macrovessels, then µ for microvessels. *Output :* expressed as velocity of red cells in cm per sec.

Microvessels position

Vessel	Diameter (cm then µ)	Muscle	Nerves	Output (cm/sec)
Aorta (arch)	2 to 3			60
Aorta	1 to 2			30
Arterioles	100 to 40	CML[+++]	Symp+++	0.5
Pre-capill. art.	30	CML[+]	0	0.5
Capillaries	10 to 5	O	0	0.005
	(50 % 4.5			
Post-capill. venulae	20 to 30	0	0	0.01
Venules	40 to 100	CML[+]	Symp[+]	0.2 to 0.5
Veins	0.5 to 1			15 to 20
Vena cava	3			10 to 15

(30 to 40 µ) or pre-capillary sphincters associated with smooth muscle cells which are not, however, innervated (Wiedeman, 1981); true capillaries (10 to 5 µ, 50 %< 4.5 µ) with a less elaborate structure; post-capillary venules (20 to 30 µ) surrounded by pericytes with few smooth muscle cells, venules (40 to 100 µ) with few parietal smooth muscle cells and little innervation. A fundamental feature of the microvessels is their low rate of blood flow compared to systemic vessels. The lowest flow rates are found in the post-capillary venules, producing the lowest shear forces in the whole vascular tree.

The various components of the microcirculation unit have specialized functions *(Table II)*, which confer a certain functional coherence to the system. The well-innervated terminal arterioles represent the organ of perfusion of

Table 2. The «microcirculatory unit» (JF Merlen). Functional specific role for each group of microvessels.

Microcirculatory unit

100	▶ 50 à 30 µ	Arterioles Pre-capillaries arterioles	Tissue perfusion Systemic blood pressure
	10 to 5 µ	Capillaries	Interstitial tissue exchange (gas and liquids)
	20 to 30 µ	Post-capillaries venulae	Cell transit to tissues (blood cells thoroughfare)
100	◀ 40 µ	Venulae	Venous blood reservoir Venous pressure

M.R. *Boisseau*

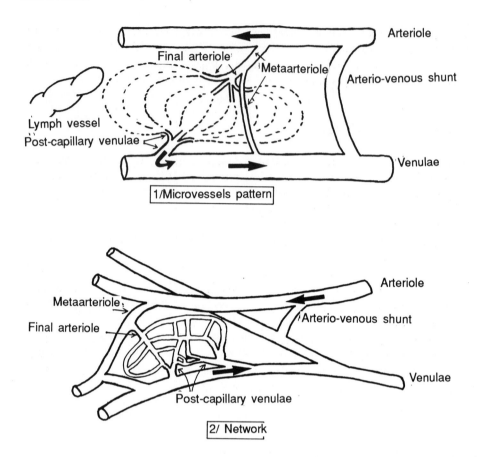

Figure 1. Schematic draft of the microcirculation. Adaptability of the network. Aspects related to microvessels of skeletal muscles.

the unit, and are the main source of peripheral resistance which is a significant regulator of blood pressure. Metabolic and mechanical regulation of the unit take place in the precapillary arterioles which adjust to alterations in arteriolar perfusion. Interstitial exchanges occur essentially in the capillaries, although water and some molecules also exchange with tissues in the venules. The postcapillary venules are an important site of cellular exchanges, and the main point of entry of leucocytes into tissues. Finally, the venules have a capacitance function in the blood reservoir. The exchange of water and small molecules between the venules and tissues can lead to a build up of venous pressure in some circumstances (orthostatic venous hyperpressure for example).

It can thus be seen there is a relationship between structure and function of the various components of the microcirculation unit. Although there are differences in the arrangement of these components in the various organs, their functions are invariably in the above-mentioned sequence.

Anatomy and Histology

The first anatomical and histological descriptions of the blood vessels go back to Harvey (1578-1657) and Malpighi (1628-1694). In recent years, the structures of microvessels have been described in detail for the various organs of the body [39, 44, 77, 85]. Without entering into details, a few essential points are worth mentioning here.

The innervation of arterioles stops at the terminal arterioles, but is extended by extra-vascular fibers.

The true capillaries have a simple mono-cellular architecture whose structure varies from organ to organ. It is fenestrated in parenchyma, discontinuous in hematopoietic organs, but continuous in skin, skeletal muscles and the nervous system.

An important anatomical feature is the presence of arteriovenous anastomoses whose shunting action is central to microcirculatory function. These anastomoses form a linked network with considerable adaptive properties. *Figure 1* shows a typical network in skeletal muscle.

Regulation of the microcirculation

Three main parameters can be regulated in the microcirculation unit. *Blood flow* is influenced by both local and general control systems. *Exchanges* with interstitial tissue and lymphatics, and *cell transit* involving rheological processes are all subjected to a number of controlling influences.

Regulation of flow and pressure

General factors

The neurohormonal regulation (baroreflexes) is coordinated by bareoreceptors situated in the aorta and carotid sinus. Neurohormones (adrenaline and noradrenaline) bind to alpha-1 post-synaptic receptors on smooth muscle cells of the terminal arterioles, opening calcium channels and allowing Ca^{2+} ions to enter cells. Post-synaptic alpha-2 and beta receptors also play a role, and several other hormonal systems exert an influence on microvessels [30], such as :

- angiotensin II (renin-angiotensin II-aldosterone system) which has a vasoconstrictor and stabilizing action;

- vasopressin (antidiuretic hormone) which responds to signals from the baroreceptors;

- the vasodilator action of kinin from the kallicrein-kinin-bradykinin system.

Endothelial cells regulate vessel diameter (bore size) and so influence both blood flow and pressure in a complex battery of mechanisms. A principle action is mediated by secretion of endothelium-derived relaxing factor (EDRF) discovered by Fruchgott, and identified as nitrogen dioxide [60]. The endothelium in turn interacts with neurohormones in a complex manner [78]. The following actions have been identified : inactivation of bradykinin, conversion of angiotensin I to II by converting enzyme, secretion of the vasoconstrictor endothelin and the vasodilator prostacyclin. All these actions impinge on parietal smooth muscle cells. The endothelium can thus be seen as an important effector organ for the regulation of blood flow in the microcirculation. It also modulates the shearing forces between blood and vessel walls (stress regulation).

Local factors

Locally acting mechanisms have particular importance at the terminal arterioles which are devoid of innervation, and so are less sensitive to the influences described above. There are considerable differences, though, from one organ to another. A reduction in oxygen partial pressure (PO_2) leads to a relaxation of smooth muscle cells, and hence vasodilatation. The main mediator here is adenosine. However, cerebral blood flow is not affected by this mechanism, but reacts rather to P_{CO2} and H^+ ion concentration.

The myogenic reflex is triggered by stretching of smooth muscle cells (stretch activation) leading to vasoconstriction, especially in response to hyperpressure on the venous side of the microcirculatory unit. Various mediators have been identified including : a cellular sensor, endothelin and PO_2.

Another property of the microcirculation has been described recently by Intaglietta [37], which he refers to as vasomotion. It consists of cycles of vasoconstriction and vasodilation mainly occurring in arterioles originating in the forks of the microvessels (pace-maker effect). This activity is increased in certain metabolic and hemodynamic stress states. Loss of this property appears to be detrimental to tissue perfusion.

Finally, the contractions of lymphatic saccules also play a part in the local control of blood flow in the microcirculation.

Regulation of tissue exchange

The overall perfusion in the microcirculation unit depends on the resultant of the residual motor pressure and the extent of vasoconstriction of the terminal arterioles and precapillary arterioles (precapillary sphincters). The terminal arterioles are responsive to general influences, whereas the capillaries are more sensitive to local factors. Blood flow in the microcirculatory network can thus vary considerably from one territory to another, and in some areas permanent or temporary shut-down of the microcirculation can occur. This is frequently observed in muscles and skin where such processes represent an essential mechanism of regulation of volume and pressure in the arterial system. The venous side has more effect on blood volume via the blood storage properties of the venules. The arteriolar side via its vasomotor properties has more effect on pressure.

Exchange of gases, fluid and molecules between the blood and tissues is an essential property of the microcirculation unit. The alteration in hemodynamics in these tiny vessels (see below) leads to the formation of a slow moving circumferential layer of plasma, which favors exchange of substances between blood and tissues. This plasma layer is observed in nearly all vessels, but has particular importance in two vessel types :

- in the true capillaries where exchanges with tissues occur first with the plasma layer, and then as the bore narrows, with plasma and cells in contact with vessel walls (50 % of capillaries have a diameter below (5 μ). Exchange of gases takes place principally on the contact of red cells with vessel walls. These cells move in single file or in *rouleaux* in these narrow vessels. The capillary system is particularly sensitive to the perfusion pressure, and thus to arteriolar vasomotricity;

- venules where the sluggish flow favors exchanges between the plasma layer and tissues. Venous hyperpressure will clearly have an influence on this process.

Exchanges are therefore regulated essentially by pressure with an equilibrium between hydrostatic and oncotic pressures at the vessel wall *(Figure 2)*. Proper functioning of the lymphatic system is also required, with collection of fluid from atria and vesicles with their 3-6 per minute cyclic contractions.

Regulation of cellular exchange (microrheology)

Alteration in local hemodynamics

The Fahraeus effect is a characteristic property of the microcirculation, wich is manifest in vessels with diameters below 100 μ. Initially is characterized by a fall in hematocrit, which is much lower in microvessels. Blood flow

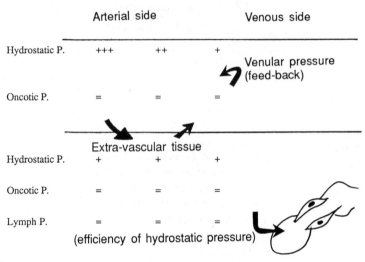

Figure 2. Tissue exchange : role of different pressures. Importance of a low pressure in the venulae.

is characterized by a central arrangement of red cells in discontinuous *rouleaux* separated by white cells and surrounded by a circumferential plasma layer which contains a significant proportion of platelets. Except in the true capillaries, this layer moves more slowly than the inner red cell stream which favors the restoration of a normal hematocrit at the output of the micro-circulation [26]. The fall in hematocrit reduces viscosity, although this is sometimes increased by sedimentation and accumulation [25].

Leucocytes tend to move to the circumference in the plasma layer under chemotactic influences. In fact, the microcirculation appears to be the major site of action of leucocytes since blood flow is relatively slow, and is even further slowed as it meanders through the network [45]. The formation of *rouleaux* and aggregates of red cells further enhances the centrifugal move-ment of leucocytes [25].

There are, however, considerable regional differences in blood flow in the microcirculation in both normal and pathological circumstances. There is often and uneven distribution of cells at the vessel forks, and plasma tends to pass into the branch with the lower flow (plasma skimming effect) [65].

In the presence of hyperfibrinogenemia, for example, the increased aggre-gation of red cells with further hamper flow at vessel forks. In addition, it will favor stasis, especially in the post-capillary venules increasing the centrifugal movement of white cells and accelerating the passage of fluid across the vessel walls into tissues [26].

Behavior of blood cells

In order to pass through true capillaries, red cells must change their shape. Cell deformability depends on three factors : overall shape, membrane viscoelasticity and viscosity of cell contents. These parameters may be altered in various pathologies, the most notable being sickle cell anemia and diabetes. Leucocytes are 100 times more rigid than red cells [73], and can thus clog vessels with diameters under 20 μ. Normally, unlike red cells, they pass through arteriovenous anastomoses at a relatively high rate, which means that the microcirculation contains lower levels of white cells than does the general circulation [26]. However, a completely different situation arises under inflammatory conditions, when white cells move to the circumference of vessels tending to roll slowly along vessel walls. White cells normally only pass into tissues from the postcapillary venules. This is where flow is most sluggish and shear rates are lowest. Hematocrit is on the increase and may rise above normal due to sedimentation and accumulation. The mean velocity of leucocytes is at its lowest ebb in these vessels, and polymorphonuclear neutrophils (PMN), monocytes and lymphocytes readily move to the circumference and migrate across vessel walls thereby entering tissues.

These findings have important clinical implications. Under pathological conditions giving rise to venous hyperpressure or inflammation, white cells adhere and become activated on contact with vessel walls in the postcapillary venules and venules. White cells are sensitive to shear, and will only adhere if the shear-stress with the vessel walls is under 5 dynes/cm^2 [40], which is encountered in vessels where flow rates are low.

Endothelial cells and cellular adhesion

The endothelium has a normal hemostatic action mediated by an assortment of substances such as the platelet anti-aggregant, prostacyclin (PGI2), thrombomodulin which neutralizes thrombin, plasminogen activator (t-PA), and heparan sulfate which binds to antithrombin III. On the other hand, the endothelium can exhibit prothrombotic activity abetted by the presence of cytokines (IL1, IL6, TNF) and pathological factors such as oxygen-derived free radicals. The following processes have been described :

- alteration in the shape of endothelial cells, with the protruding cells forming gaps between cells [26];
- expression of integrins [15], ligands for leucocytes such as ICAM (lymphocytes), ILAM-1 (Polymorphonuclear and monocytes) and GMP-140 released from granules and expressed on the cell surface [28];
- secretion of a tissue factor, triggering the extrinsic coagulation pathway (factor VII pathway); secretion of von Willebrand factor, a red cell ligand [75,76]; PAI-1; platelet activating factor (PAF) [67]; interleukin 1 (IL1);

25

- reduction in anti-thrombotic activities.

In response to these changes, leucocytes adhere to and interact with the endothelium. The nature of these interactions which has only recently been uncovered appear to have considerable pathophysiological significance [34, 42].

Leucocyte activation is stimulated by :

- the presence of cytokine : Interleukin1, Interleukin6, tumor necrosis factor (TNF) [61];

- chemoattractants FLMP [51], C5a;

- agonists ADP [3], endotoxins, LTB4 with a direct action on PMN [51, 59], PAF [16, 67, 79];

- thrombin [80].

Activation is characterized biochemically by the expression of leu-CAM beta-integrins (CD11/CD18) [2, 61].

Interactions with endothelium are favored by stasis, and so tend to occur mainly in the post-capillary venules. The regulation of these processes is poorly understood, but 13-HODE and 23-HETES [7] are throught to have a stabilizing action, one with an activating and the other a deactivating effect. In addition, leucocytes appear to secrete their own adhesion inhibitor, LAI [84].

Activated monocytes in contact with the endothelium have enhanced procoagulant properties, secreting a tissue factor and expressing binding sites for fibrinogen and factors Xa and VIIa [1, 74] and PGE2 [72].

Red cells may also adhere to activated endothelium with von Willebrand factor as possible ligand [75].

Amplification in pathology

A whole repertoire of cell-mediated processes underlie the interactions between white cells and endothelium. For example, endothelial cells secrete PAF [13], and IL1. PMN produce PAF [69] and cathepsin G which also acts on platelets. The combination of cathepsin G and granulocyte elastase degrades heparin cofactor II, which then exhibits strong chemoattractant properties [36]. Amplification of LTB4 production by PMN is triggered by erythrocyte LTA4 [46, 71]. Platelets produce PAF and ADP which acts on PMN and other platelets. Monocytes produce PAF, IL1 and NAF [14]. Lastly, lymphocyte LIF influences adhesion of PMN [64].

It can be seen, therefore, that there is a strong link between ischemia and thrombosis. In ischemia, PMN activate endothelial cells via production of free radicals [41], and can bind factor Xa and fibrinogen to CR3 receptors [86]. They also have a vasoconstrictor action of the endothelium. Endothelial cells can bind factor Xa and produce fibrin, a property shared by monocytes. Various pathological conditions, of which diabetes is a prime example, stimulate these processes [66].

Such mechanisms play a crucial role in ischemia (PMN/endothelial interactions) and thrombosis (monocytes/endothelium/factor VII interactions) [55], and better understanding of these process will undoubtedly spur the development of new therapeutic strategies.

Investigations

Investigation of the microcirculation

In clinical practice, investigations are aimed at exploration of the structure and function of microvessels. In vasospastic disorders (Raynaud's syndrome, scleroderma), diabetes, and hypertension, the structure of the microvessels can be studied by periungual or conjunctival capillaroscopy along with the fluorescein permeability tests. This can be combined with digital plethysmography where the arterial pressure in the digits is measured before and after venous counterpressure.

In chronic arteriopathy of lower limbs, residual function of microvessels, especially after ischemia, can be explored by Doppler-Laser photometry which determines the flow rate of blood cells in a 1 mm^3 volume under the skin. Transcutaneous measurement of PO_2 is also employed. Determination of subcutaneous transit of labelled substances can be used to evaluate impairment of permeability and the origin of edema.

Investigation of microrheology

Direct investigation of blood cells has mostly been carried out in animals, and is not yet really feasible in man. Three main types of investigation have been employed.

Analysis of rheological factors in zones of stasis

Measurement of viscosity at low shear rates, which assesses the effects of aggregation of red cells, can give an *in vitro* estimate of potential rates of blood flow in post-capillary venules as well as in zones of stasis such as the vessels immediately after a stenosis or in ischemic regions. Such investigations are of value prior to surgical treatment of arteriopathy of the lower limbs, and in disorders of the venous system.

Deformability of blood cells

The deformability of red cells and leucocytes can be evaluated *ex vivo*, and has been the subject of a considerable body of research. There are marked

27

an consistent alterations in erythrocyte deformability in sickle cell anemia, xerocytosis and poorly controlled diabetes, although in vascular disease, they are not so well established. Furthermore, the effects of the alteration in deformability are not easy to assess *in vivo*. For example, in sickle cell anemia, the decrease in deformability appears to have less pathological significance than the adhesion of cells to activated vessel walls, although it is clear that the two phenomena are related.

Leucocytes remain rigid after activation [5], and the reduced deformability of these cells has been implicated in some manifestations of vascular disease [52, 53].

Methods for analyzing cellular deformability such as timing passage through filters of graded pore size are not always interpretable as aggregates of cells can plug filter pores. This has now given rise to the notion of cellular filterability rather than deformability. The value of ektacytometry has also been questioned due to the extraphysiological conditions under which it is used, and its extreme sensitivity to intracellular viscosity.

Leucocyte activation

Methods for the evaluation of PMN and monocyte activation are being developed, and when available should throw more light on the role of these cells in ischemia and thrombosis. In the absence of acute inflammatory processes, plasma levels of elastase and myeloperoxidase are related to activation of PMN. The determination of the expression of leu-CAM beta-integrins on membranes can give an estimate of the proportion of activated circulating leucocytes (MAC 1, CR 3) [15]. Polymerization of actin [5, 23, 58], also reflects the state of activation or priming of leucocytes.

Another approach is to assess activation of coagulation at the surface of monocytes, by determination of factor Xa, the presence of derivatives of fibrin, and fibrinogen receptors [38, 43, 56].

The estimation of ischemia and thrombotic risk will undoubtedly benefit from further developments in these areas. From a pharmacological point of view, drugs acting on the endothelium and leucocytes and the interactions between them could then be devised [23].

Pathophysiology

Diseases of the microcirculation have a variety of causes, involving damage to the structure of, and impairments in vasomotricity of the microvessels. Rheological factors are involved to differing extents in such disorders, and much remains to be found out about their pathophysiological significance. However, they appear to be implicated in four main types of pathology.

Vasospastic disorders

Raynaud's syndrome is essentially a disorder of vasomotricity, and rheological parameters are usually normal in this condition. However, in acrocyanosis, acrosyndromes secondary to risk factors and in scleroderma, microrheological factors play a role in the inflammatory syndrome.

High blood pressure

Essential hypertension can be viewed as a model of abnormal pressure and flow regulation in terminal arterioles. The advent of calcium blockers in the treatment of high blood pressure has highlighted the role of peripheral resistance under this condition. High blood pressure is accompanied by an increase in plasma viscosity due to the raised fibrinogen levels and the hyperaggregation of red cells. These disorders illustrate the significance of the microcirculation unit, not only for its resistive properties, but also for the balance between rheological and plasma factors within microvessels.

Rheological diseases

Red cell diseases

Sickle cell anemia is characterized by a disorder in deformability of red cells, also observed in the heterozygotes. It is due to cellular dehydration, and an increased intra-cellular hemoglobin concentration, enhanced by attachment of hemoglobin S granules to the plasma membrane. In fact, this defect in deformability appears less deleterious than the increased tendency of these altered red cells to adhere to the damaged or activated endothelium giving rise to microvascular thromboses.

Hereditary familial xerocytosis is characterized by a dehydration of red cells due to a massive influx of Ca^{2+} ions. This rheological disorder resulting from an increase in intracellular viscosity is readily visualized by ektacytometry.

Hyperviscosity syndromes

Various syndromes of plasma or erythrocyte hyperviscosity secondary to hematological diseases such as Vaquez polyglobulia and dysproteinemias have been described. In shock, there is a massive adhesion of leucocytes to the endothelium especially in the adult respiratory distress syndrome (ARDS) [63].

Mention should also be made of the primary hyperviscosity syndromes, largely idiopathic, which are revealed by an impairment of the microcirculation especially in the inner ear with repercussions on hearing. In this case, there is a chronic contraction of plasma volume, sometimes accompanied by elevations in hematocrit and fibrinogen. The mechanism is poorly understood, although it impairs the microcirculation. It may have some relation to hypertension since calcium blockers and drugs which reduce peripheral resistance improve the condition.

Vascular diseases and microcirculation

Disorders of the microcirculation are fundamental to vascular disease both from a pathophysiological and therapeutic standpoint.

Venous disease

Chronic superficial venous insufficiency induces a progressive impairment in the microcirculation on the venous side, leading to venous hyperpressure [8]. The venules are the sites of disorders of permeability, resulting in edema, contraction of plasma volume with concomitant hyperviscosity and enhanced aggregation of red cells. These initially local disorders tend to become disseminated throughout the circulation. Progressive inhibition of flow in post-capillary venules also favors adhesion of leucocytes and ulceration.

Arterial disease

Atherosclerosis, an inflammatory and deforming disease of arterial walls, is accompanied by generalized rheological disorders. Risk factors for atheroma such as high blood pressure and diabetes [38] tend to induce bouts of inflammation accompanied by increased secretion of cytokines. The rheological disturbances can be largely accounted for by the hyperfibrinogenemia, the contraction of plasma volume stemming from the enhanced vascular permeability and the activation of leucocytes and endothelial cells [20]. In addition, abnormalities in membrane lipids [23] decrease the deformability and enhance the priming of circulating cells. A variety of compensatory mechanisms tend to conceal the rheological disorders which only become apparent where there is a defect in driving pressure and flow in the large systemic vessels harboring atherosclerotic plaques. Three areas tend to be affected :

- zones of stenosis : platelets are activated around plaques essentially as a result of shear stress. In the stagnant post-stenosed zone, the low flow rates favor adhesion of leucocytes to the activated endothelium thereby triggering coagulation [19];

- post-stenosis ischemic zones : the initial studies of Bagge [4, 5], Engler [17] and Gaethgens [27] have demonstrated adhesion of leucocytes to the endothelium in ischemic vessels. This significant phenomenon blocks the microcirculation (no-reflow effect) [31, 35, 53] via local diffusion of cytokines and free radicals, and especially LTB4 [29]. Vasomotor disorders thus develop in parallel with the ischemia [32];

- peri-thrombotic zones : adherence of cells to vessel walls in peri-thrombotic regions also tends to aggravate the lesions.

Coronary disease and myocardial infarction also lead to rheological disorders [18]. One index of infarction is represented by the leucocyte count [24, 33, 87], but it can also be assessed from the adhesive properties of these cells [70], and their state of activation [47]. The rigidity of leucocytes indicated by filtration tests is related to their degree of activation [12, 54]. In animal studies, depletion or inactivation of leucocytes using monoclonal antibodies has been shown to reduce the area of ischemia [57, 62, 68].

Activation and rheological changes in leucocytes are also observed in stroke [11, 21, 22, 81, 83].

Thus it can be seen that although the microrheological alterations may not be the cause of the vascular obstruction from atheroma or platelet aggregation, they do tend to make the situation worse [10]. Besides platelet behavior and vasomotor factors, rheological factors do, therefore, need to be taken into account in such conditions.

Thrombosis

Microrheological factors play a dual role in thrombotic processes. A thrombus can form on damaged and activated endothelium in zones where blood flow is low. The coagulant properties of blood cells, especially those of monocytes may be translocated, inducing venous thromboses [19, 55, 56] or disseminated intravascular coagulation [43].

Conclusion

The microcirculation is regulated in a complex manner by a combination of vasomotor and flow control mechanisms. The characteristics of the microcirculation vary from territory to territory and from organ to organ, but its role in a number of pahtological processes is now beginning to be unravelled.

31

Microrheology is intimately bound up with the microcirculation in both health and disease, and is receiving increasing attention in view of its relationship with inflammatory processes and microcirculatory hemodynamics. The characteristics of blood flow in the microvessels thus represents a potential target for new therapeutic agents, especially those designed for the treatment and prevention of vascular disease.

References

1. Altieri DC, Bader R, Mannuci PM *et al.* Oligospecificity of the cellular adhesion receptor MAC-1 encompasses an inducible recognition specificity for fibrinogen. J Cell Biol, 1988; 107 : 1893-1900.

2. Arnaout MA. Structure and function of the leukocyte adhesion molecules CD11/CD18. Blood, 1990; 75 : 1037-1050.

3. Axtell RA, Sandborg RR, Smolen JE *et al.* Exposure of human neutrophils to exogenous nucleotides causes elevation in intracellular calcium, transmembrane calcium fluxes and an alteration of a cytosolic factor resulting in enhanced superoxyde production in response to FLMP and arachidonic acid Blood, 1990; 75 : 1324-1332.

4. Bagge U, Amundson B, Lauritzen C. White blood cells deformability and plugging of skeletal muscle capillaries in haemorrhagic shock. Acta Physiol Scand, 1980; 108 : 159-163.

5. Bagge U. Granulocyte rheology. Blood Cells, 1976; 2 : 481-490.

6. Belloc F, Vincendeau P, Freyburger G *et al.* A flow cytometry study of the activation of polymorphonuclear cells. J Leuk Biol, (in press).

7. Buchanan MR, Bastida E. Endothelium and underlying membrane reactivity with platelets, leukocytes and tumor cells : regulation by the lipoxygenase-derived fatty acid metabolites, 13-HODE and HETES. Med Hypotheses, 1988; 27 : 317-325.

8. Chabanel A, Glacet-Bernard A, Lelong F, *et al.* Increased blood cell aggregation in retinal vein occlusion. Br J Haemat, 1990; 75 : 127-131.

9. Casillas JM, Didier JP, Lucet A *et al.* Adaptation cardio-respiratoire, métabolique et microcirculatoire au cours de l'artériopathie oblitérante des membres inférieurs. Sem Hôp Paris, 1990; 66 : 333-337.

10. Ciufetti G, Mercuri M, Rizzo MT *et al.* Human leukocyte rheology and tissue ischaemia. Eur J Clin Invest, 1989; 19 : 323-327.

11. Ciuffetti G, Mercuri M, Mannarino E *et al.* Leucocyte rheology in the early stages of ischaemic stroke. Klin Wochenschr, 1989; 67 : 762-763.

12. Ciuffetti G, Bellomo G, Mercuri M *et al.* Leucocyte rheology in controlled coronary ischaemia. Int J Cardiol, 1989; 193-198.

13. Coëffier E, Delautier D, Le Couedic JP *et al.* Cooperation between platelets and neutrophils for PAF-acether (Platelet-activating Factor) formation. J Leuk Biol, 1990; 47 : 23-243.

14. Colditz I, Zwahlen R, Dewald B, Baggiolini M. *In vivo* inflammatory activity of neutrophil-activating factor, novel chemotactic peptide derived from human monocytes. Amer. J. Pathol., 1989; 134 : 755-760.

15. Detmers PA, Wright SD. Adhesion-promoting receptors of leukocytes. Current Op. Immunol., 1988; 1 : 10-15.

16. Dillon PK, Fitzpatrick MF, Ritter AB *et al.* Effect of platelet-activating factor on leukocyte adhesion to microvascular endothelium. Inflammation, 1988; 12 : 563-570.

17. Engler RL, Schmidt-Schönbein GW, Pavelee RS. Leukocyte capillary plugging in myocardial ischaemia and reperfusion in the dog. Am J Pathol, 1983; 111 : 98-111.

18. Engler RL, Dahlgreen MD, Peterson MA *et al.* Accumulation of polymorphonuclear leukocytes during experimental myocardial ischemia. Heart Circ Physiol, 1986; 20 : H93-H100.

19. Ernst E, Hammerschmidt DE, Bagge U *et al.* Leukocytes and the risk of ischaemic diseases. JAMA, 1987; 257 : 2318-2324.

20. Enrst E, Matrai A. Altered red and white blood cell rheology in type II diabetes. Diabetes, 1986; 35 : 1412-1415.

21. Ernst E, Matrai A, Paulsen F. Leukocyte rheology in recent stroke. Stroke, 1987; 18 : 59-62.

22. Ernst E, Matrai A, Marshall M. Blood rheology in patients with transient ischemic attacks. Stroke, 1988; 19 : 634-636.

23. Freyburgher G, Gin H, Heape A *et al.* Phospholipid and fatty acid composition of erythrocytes in type I and type II diabetes. Metabolism, 1989; 38 : 673-678.

24. Friedman GD, Klatsky AL, Siegelaub AB. The leukocyte count at a predictor of myocardial infarction. N Engl J Med, 1974; 290 : 1275-1278.

25. Gaethghens P. Microvascular flow disturbances : rheological aspects. In Manabe H *et al.,* Microcirculation in circulatory disorders. Springer Verlag, 1988.

26. Gaethgens P. Pathways and interactions of white cells in the microcirculation. In K Messmert *et al.,* Progress in applied microcirculation. Karger, 1987.

27. Gaethgens SP, Ley K, Pries AR *et al.* Actual interaction between leukocytes and microvascular blood flow. Prog Appl Microcirc, 1985; 7 : 15-28.

28. Geng JG, Bevilacqua MP, Moore KL *et al.* Rapid neutrophil adhesion to activated endothelium mediated by GMP-140. Nature, 1990; 343 : 757-758.

29. Goldman G, Welbourn R, Paterson IS *et al.* Ischemia-induced neutrophil activation and diapedesis is lipoxygenase dependent. Surgery, 1990; 107 : 428-433.

30. Granger HJ, Schelling ME, Lewis RE *et al.* Physiology and pathobiology of the microcirculation. Am J Otolaryngol, 1988; 9 : 264-277.

31. Granger DN, Benoit JN, Suzuki M *et al.* Leukocyte adherence to venular endothelium during ischemia-reperfusion. Am J Physiol, 1989; 257 : G683-G688.

32. Grossman HJ, Zambetis M. Leucocyte-induced endothelium-dependent vasodilatation and post-ischaemic vasospasm in the isolated rat superior mesenteric artery. Br J Exp Path, 1989; 70 : 515-523.

33. Haines AP, Howarth D, North WRS *et al.* Haemostatic variables and the outcome of myocardial infarction. Thromb. Haemostas, 1983; 50 : 800-803.

34. Harlan JM. Leukocyte-endothelial interactions. Blood, 1985; 65 : 513-525.

35. Hernandez LA, Grisham MB, Twohig B *et al.* Role of neutrophils in ischemia-reperfusion-induced microvascular injury. Am J Physiol, 1987; 253 : H699-H703.

36. Hoffman M, Pratt CW, Brown RL *et al*. Heparin cofactor II-proteinase reaction products exhibit neutrophil chemoattractant activity. Blood, 1989; 73 : 1682-1685.
37. Intaglietta M. Vasomotion and flow modulation in the microcirculation. *In Progress in applied microcirculation* Vol 15. M Intaglietta Ed, 1 Vol, Karger 1989.
38. Jude B, Watel A, Fontaine O *et al*. Distinctive feature of procoagulant response of monocytes from diabetic patients. Haemostasis, 1989; 19 : 65-73.
39. Larcan A. *In Microcirculation et hémorhéologie*. A Larcan, JF Stoltz, Eds, 1 Vol, Masson 1970.
40. Lawrence MB, Smith CW, Eskin SG *et al*. Effect of venous shear stress on CD18-mediated neutrophil adhesion to cultured endothelium. Blood, 1990; 75 : 227-237.
41. Lewis MS, Whatley RE, Cain P *et al*. Hydrogen peroxide stimulates the synthesis of platelet activating factor by endothelium and induces endothelial cell-dependent neutrophil adhesion. J. Clin Invest, 1988; 82 : 2045-2055.
42. Lipowsky HH, House SD, Firrell JC. Leukocyte endothelium adhesion and microvascular hemodynamics. Adv Exp Med Biol, 1988; 242 : 85-93.
43. Luscher E. Activated leukocytes and the haemostatic system. Rev. Inf. Diseases, 1987; 9 : 5546-5557.
44. Manabe BW. Microcirculation in circulatory disorders. Manabe H, Zweifach BW, Messmer K Eds, 1 Vol. Springer-Verlag, 1988.
45. Mayrowitz HN, Kang SJ, Herscovici B *et al*. Leukocyte adherence initiation in skeletal muscle capillaries and venules. Microvasc Res, 1987; 33 : 22-34.
46. McGee JE, Fitzpatrick FA. Erythrocyte-neutrophil interactions : formation of leukotriene B4 by transcellular biosynthesis. Proc Natl Acad Sci USA, 1986; 83 : 1349-1353.
47. Mehta J. Dinerman J, Mehta P *et al*. Neutrophil function in ischemic heart disease. Circulation, 1989; 79 : 549-556.
48. Messmer K, Hammersen F. Microcirculation and inflammation : vessel wall-inflammatory cells-mediator interaction. *In Progress in applied microcirculation*, vol 12. Messmer Ed, 1 Vol Karger, 1987.
49. Messmer K, Hammersen. Cerebral microcirculation. In Progress in applied microcirculation vol 16, Messmer K, Hammersen F Eds, 1 Vol Karger, 1990.
50. Mortillaro NA. The physiology and pharmacology of the microcirculation, Vol 1. N. Mortillaro A. Ed., 1 Vol. Academic Press, 1983.
51. Nagai K, Katori M. Possible changes in the leukocyte membrane as a mechanism of leukocyte adhesion to the venular walls induced by leukotrien B4 and FLMP in the microvasculature of the hamster cheek pouch. Int. Microcirc J Clin Exp, 1988; 7 : 305-314.
52. Nash GB, Jones JG, Mikita J *et al*. Methods and theory for analysis of flow of white cell subpopulations through micropore filters. Brit Haemat J, 1988; 70 : 165-170.
53. Nash GB, Thomas PRS, Dormandy JA. Abnormal flow properties of white blood cells in patients with severe ischaemia of the leg. Brit Med J, 1988; 296-302.
54. Nash GB, Christopher B, Morris AJR *et al*. Changes in the flow properties of white cells after acute myocardial infarction. Br Heart J, 1989; 62 : 329-334.
55. Nygaard OP, Unneberg K, Reikeras O, Osterud B. Thromboplastin activity of blood monocytes after hip replacement. Scand J Clin Lab Invest, 1990; 50 : 183-186.
56. Ollivier V, Sheibani A, Chollet-Martin S *et al*. Monocyte procoagulant activity and membrane-associated D-Dimer after knee replacement surgery. Thromb Res, 1989; 55 : 179-185.

57. O'Neill PG, Charlat ML, Michael LH *et al.* Influence of neutrophil depletion on myocardial function and flow after reversible ischemia. Am J. Physiol, 1989; 256 : H341-H351.

58. Packman CH, Lichtman MA. Activation of neutrophils : measurement of actin conformational changes by flow cytometry. Blood cells, 1990; 16.

59. Palmblad J, Lindström P, Lerner R. Leukotrien B4 induced hyperadhesiveness of endothelial cells for neutrophils. Bioch Bioph Res Comm, 1990; 166 : 848-851.

60. Palmer RMJ, Ferrige AG, Moncada S. Nitric oxide release accounts for the biological activity of endothelium-derived relaxing factor. Nature, 1987; 327 : 524-526.

61. Pober JS. Cytoline-mediated activation of vascular endothelium. Am J. Pathol, 1988; 133 : 426-433.

62. Romson JL, Hook BG, Steven BS *et al.* Reduction of the extent of ischemic myocardial injury by neutrophil depletion in the dog. Circulation, 1983; 67 : 1016-1023.

63. Rossignon MD, Khayat D, Royer C *et al.* Functional and metabolic activity of polymorphonuclear leukocytes from patients with adult respiratory distress syndrome : results of a randomized double-blind placebo-controlled study on the activity of prostaglandin E1. Anesthesiology, 1990; 72 : 276-281.

64. Schainberg H, Borish L, King M *et al.* Leukocyte inhibitory factor stimulates neutrophil-endothelial cell adhesion. J. Immunol. 1988; 141 : 3055-3060.

65. Secomb TW, Fleischman GF, Papenfuss HD *et al.* Effects of reduced perfusion and hematocrit on flow distribution in capillary networks. In Messmer K, ref. 48, pp 205-211.

66. Setiadi H, Wautier JL, Courillon-Mallet A *et al.* Increased adhesion to fibronectin and MO-1 expression by diabetic monocytes. J Immunol., 1987; 138 : 3230-3234.

67. Shalit M, Dabiri GA, Southwick FS. Platelet-activating factor both stimulates and «primes» human polymorphonuclear leukocyte actin filament assembly. Blood, 1987; 70 : 1921-1927.

68. Simpson PJ, Todd III RF, Fantone JC *et al.* Reducation of experimental canine myocardial reperfusion injury by a monoclonal antibody (anti-Mol, anti-CD11b) that inhibits leukocyte adhesion. J Clin Invest, 1988; 81 : 624-629.

69. Sisson JH, Prescott SM, McIntyre TM *et al.* Production of platelet-activating factor by stimulated human polymorphonuclear leukocytes. J Immunol, 1987; 138 : 3918-3926.

70. Smith BD, Thomas JL, Gillespie JA. Abnormal erythrocyte endothelial adherence in ischemic heart disease. Clin Hemorh, 1990; 10 : 241-253.

71. Stern A, Serhan CN. Human red cells enhance the formation of 5-lipoxygenase-derived products by neutrophils. Free Rad Res Comms, 1989; 7 : 335-339.

72. Takayama TK, Miller C, Szabo G. Elevated tumor necrosis factor production concomitant to elevated prostaglandin E2 production by trauma patients' monocytes. Arch Surg, 1990; 125 : 29-35.

73. Thompson TN, La celle PL, Cokelet GR. Perturbation of red blood cell flow in small tubes by white blood cells. Pflügers Arch, 1989; 413 : 372-377.

74. Trezzini C, Jungi TW, Kuhnert P *et al.* Fibrinogen association with human monocytes : evidence for constitutive expression of fibrinogen receptors and for involvement of MAC-1 (CD18, CR3) in the binding. Bioch Bioph Res Comms, 1988; 156 : 477-484.

75. Tsai HM, Sussman II, Nagel RL *et al.* Desmopressin induces adhesion of normal human erythrocytes to the endothelial surface of a perfused microvascular preparation. Blood, 1990; 75 : 261-265.

76. Tsai HM, Nagel RL, Hachter VB *et al*. Multimeric composition of endothelial cell-derived von Willebrand factor. Blood, 1989; 73 : 2074-2076.

77. Tsuchiya M. Microcirculation. An update, Vol 1. M Tsuchiya, Asano M, Mishima Y, Oda M. Eds. 1 Vol., Excerpta Medica 1987.

78. Vanhoutte PM. Endothelium and control of vascular function. Hypertension, 1989, 13, 658-667.

79. Vercellotti GM, Yin HQ, Gustafson KS *et al*. Platelet-activating factor primes neutrophil responses to agonists : role in promoting neutrophil-mediated endothelial damage. Blood, 1988; 71 : 1100-1107.

80. Vercellotti GM, Wickham NWR, Gustafson KS *et al*. Thrombin-treated endothelium primes neutrophil functions : inhibition by platelet-activating factor receptor antagonists. J Leuk Biol, 1989; 45 : 483-490.

81. Vermes I, Strik F. Altered leukocyte rheology in patients with chronic cerebrovascular disease. Stroke, 1988; 19 : 631-633.

82. Vicaut E. Paramètres fondamentaux dans la physiologie de la microcirculation. STV, 1990; 2 : 65-71.

83. Violi F, Rasura M, Alessandri C *et al*. Leukocyte response in patients suffering from acute stroke. Stroke, 1988; 19 : 1283-1284.

84. Wheeler ME, Luscinskas FW, Bevilacqua MP, Gimbrone Jr MA. Cultured human endothelial cells stimulated with cytokines or endotoxin produce an inhibitor of leukocyte adhesion. J Clin Invest, 1988; 82 : 1211-1218.

85. Wiedeman MP. An introduction to microcirculation, 1 vol. Wiedeman MP, Tuma RF, Mayrovitz HN, Eds Vol 1. Academic Press, 1981.

86. Wright SD, Weitz JJ, Huang AJ *et al*. Complement receptor type three (CD 11b/CD 18) of human polymorphonuclear leukocytes recognizes fibrinogen. Proc Natl Acad Sci USA, 1988; 85 : 7734-7738.

87. Zalokar JB, Richard JL, Claude JR. Leukocyte count, smoking and myocardial infarction. New Eng J Med, 1981; 304 : 465-468.

Fish oil and blood-vessel wall interactions. Eds P.M. Vanhoutte, Ph. Douste-Blazy.
John Libbey Eurotext, Paris © 1991, pp. 37-.51

4

Pathogenesis of atherosclerosis : from the lipid hypothesis to the lipoprotein hypothesis

J. Davignon

*Director Research Group on Hyperlipidemia and Atherosclerosis, Clinical
Research Institute of Montreal, Canada.*

Abstract

Numerous theories have been raised in an attempt to provide a simple unifying explanation for the pathogenesis of the atheromous plaque. It must be recognised that we
are dealing with a multi-factorial phenomenon which has its causes in a complex chain
of interactions involving the arterial wall, the environment and genes. There are many
convincing arguments to the effect that cholesterol plays a key role. It is the lipid hypothesis which has best stood the test of time, but it has gradually moved towards a "lipoprotein hypothesis". The latter takes into account increases in our knowledge over
the last decade and recognises the importance of lipoproteins, their surface apolipoproteins and composition anomalies which can confer atherogenous properties to these particles, even without hyperlipidemia. It has become clear that LDL are highly
atherogenous, that HDL have a protective role, and that the LDL/HDL (or apo B/apo
AI) correlation has a more discriminating predictive power than each of these elements
taken alone. Greater importance is today attached to lipoprotein modifications (changes
in composition, glucosylation, oxidation) which alter their interaction with receptors and
which favour their capture by the macrophages, the first step in the creation of the
spumous cells with which the atheroma originates. New research perspectives have also
been opened as a result of work on Lp (a) which would seem to link thrombogenesis
to atherogenesis; therapeutics have been adapted accordingly, following closely behind
these advances in our knowledge.

J. Davignon

Introduction

The atheroma process concerns mainly the intima of large and medium diameter arteries. It is ubiquitous and develops insidiously. It cans evolve slowly or spasmodically, and its clinical expression is rich and varied. A multiplicity of factors are involved, both in its creation , and in its development, and numerous theories have been put forward to provide a simple explanation for all its facits [1,2]. Benditt's theory of monoclonal proliferation [3] should be mentioned, being as it is compatible with a viral or oncogenic etiology. The platelet theory, originally upheld by Duguid and Rokitansky, gave rise to an elucidation of the role of platelets in the atheromatous process [4]. The injury-repair theory of Ross and his colleagues [5] emphasised the response of the arterial wall to an endothelial injury. This theory, which had to be rectified with increasing knowledge, greatly increased our understanding of atherogenesis. Our intention in this review is to pay particular attention to the lipid theory which has gradually moved towards the "lipoprotein hypothesis".

From the initial lesion to the adult plaque

The atheromous plaque is the result of a chain of interactions between the arterial wall, the environment and genetic factors [1,2]. Its creation is characterised by three essential components : endothelial damage, intimal cellular proliferation, and lipid infiltration.

The initial lesion probably takes the form of an injury to the endothelium. This can be the work of a wide range of aggressors such as hypercholesterolemia, oxidated lipoproteins, hemodynamic forces, a viral infection or some of the ingredients of cigarette smoke. They alter the permeability of the endothelium, favoring infiltration of the intima by cholesterol-bearing lipoproteins. The endothelium does not need to be bared in order for arterial wall repair mechanisms to be set in motion; a functional alteration can be sufficient [7]. The endothelial cells themselves take part in the process; they are activated by cytokines such as interleukin-1 and the tissue necrosis factor (TNF) and induce a local pro-coagulation activity together with leucocyte adhesion [8]. They also release growth factors (PDGF, FGF) which favour myo-intimal proliferation [9].

The endothelial injury, and the mobilisation of monocytes and platelets towards the lesion, induce in the intima a proliferation of both macrophages (emerging from the travelling monocytes) and smoothe muscle cells migrating from the media and assuming the characteristics of macrophages). Lipid infiltration is accompanied by the accumulation of cholesterol-gorged spumous cells giving rise to the "fatty streak". Infiltration continues and the adult plaque is characterised by necrotic tissue, fibrosis and extra-cellular lipid deposits. An inflammatory reaction is created, bringing into play immune mechanisms [10], and there is a proliferation of neovessels; ultimately all the layers of the arterial wall may be involved. The adult plaque may develop into stenosis or weaken the wall, dilating the artery. The classical complications are hemorrage, ulceration, clotting or thrombosis.

Risk factors

Numerous factors can increase individual susceptibility to atherosclerosis, trigger the process, favour or complicate its development. A wide range of "risk factors" has been compiled. A recent list contained more than 200 [11]. These may be environmental factors (tobacco consumption, a diet rich in saturated fats) or a genetic predisposition (hyperlipidemia, hypertension, diabetes). they usually act through an agent in the blood circulation (carbon monoxide, an excess of certain lipoproteins, rheological factors, toxic substances, virus) which damages the endothelium and induces plaque creation. The effects of cigarette smoking [1,2], or blood pressure [13] clearly indicate the mechanisms involved.

It is important to recognize that the evolution of the atheromatous process depends not only on the aggressor (carbon monoxide, turbulence and increased parietal stress, atherogenous lipoprotein) but also on endogenous protectors (the mobilisation of cholesterol outside the plaque) and the response of the arterial wall. Certains areas of high susceptibility are discernable *in vivo* by means of Evans blue colouring in the animal [14]. These areas are characterised by an increased permeability to certain circulating proteins (albumin, fibrinogen, ferritine), an increase in intimal cholesterol accumulation, and a high endothelial cell renewal rate. There are in addition arterial segments, such as the abdominal aorta, which are more vulnerable to the atheromatous process, because of a limited number of lamellar units and the absence of *vasa vasorum* [15, 16].

The key role of cholesterol

In 1843, Vogel demonstrated the presence of cholesterol in the atheromous plaque and, in 1913, Anitchkov and Chalatov induced atherosclerosis in the rabbit by adding purified cholesterol to the diet. Since then many observers have highlighted the key role of cholesterol in atherogenesis. [1, 2].

Experimentally, cholesterol present in the atheromous plaque has its origin in the plasma, mainly in the LDL (low density lipoproteins). Measures which increase blood cholesterol induce atherosclerosis in the animal, not only in herbivorous and susceptible species such as the rabbit, but also in omnivorous species (the pig) and the monkey. Inversely, treatment which reduces hypercholesterolemia, particularly in primates, cause the lesions to retrocede and the effect is proportional to the decrease in cholesterol concentrations [17, 18]. It is cholesterol which accumulates in the lesions, whatever the experimental model; this is true even when the atherosclerosis is induced in the normolipidemic rabbit at the point where the catheter tip comes repeatedly into contact with arterial wall [19]. Cholesterol itself can damage the endothelium, inducing mitoses and increasing its permeability [20].

In humans, epidemiological (transversal, comparative, prospective) studies have all established a close link between vascular atherosclerosis and blood cholesterol levels. The higher the cholesterol levels, the greater the risk of developing coronary disease. This subjects affected by heriditary forms of hypercholesterolemia are particularly vulnerable to atherosclerosis. In this context, familial xanthomatous homozygote hypercholesterolemia, with its precocious cardiovascular complications is particularly noteworthy. It has now been clearly established that a reduction in blood cholesterol decreases coronary risk [21, 23]. We have, moreover, see cases in which, by means of a reduction in blood cholesterol, the atheromatous plaque has been cut back, or its development retarded, both in peripheral arteries and in coronaries [28-31].

Emphasis on lipoproteins

Myocardial infarction can often occur without high cholesterol and triglyceride blood levels [32]. If cholesterol is a discriminator allowing the separation of subjects with differing degrees of cardiovascular risk [33] it loses this discriminating capability within the confines of one sub-group [34]. Progress in our knowledge of lipoprotein metabolism, and the discovery of new cardiovascular risk markers, have considerably influenced the lipid hypothesis. Interest has gradually moved from lipids to lipoproteins and apolipoproteins. Plasma cholesterol and the lipoproteins which carry it cannot be functionally disassociated. It has become clear that not all lipoproteins have the same atherogenous potential. Thus work over the last two decades has established that LDL were highly atherogenous, that HDL (high density lipoproteins) play a protective role against atherosclerosis, and that the LDL/HDL has a higher predictive capability than LDL or HDL taken separately.

LDL Atherogenicity

Two thirds of plasma cholesterol are associated with LDL and global cholesterol roughly reflects LDL levels. Thus the arguments put forward above as to the key role of cholesterol apply equally well and, more specifically, to LDL cholesterol. The animal species most susceptible to atherosclerosis carry their plasma cholesterol in association with LDL. In familial hypercholesterolemia, where there is a deficiency in the specific LDL receptor, these molecules are selectively increased and are at the origin of premature atheromatosis characterizing this disease. The consanguineous strain of the Watanabe rabbit (WHHL) with no LDL receptor on the all surface is an invaluable experimental subject which reproduces accurately the human application and illustrates the atherogenous potential of LDL [35]. Moreover a direct correlation has recently been established in man between plasma LDL cholesterol concentrations and the extent of "fatty streaks" observed on arterial walls during autopsy. This study involved children + young adults having taken part in the "Bogalusa Heart Study" and victims of accidental death [36]. The correlation remained valid down to the lowest levels of LDL cholesterol.

The protective role of HDL

The protective role of HDL is based on a series of arguments having their origins both in metabolic studies and in pathological and epidemiological observations [1, 37].
Unlike LDL, HDL dot not accumulate in the arterial wall. Animal species which resist atherosclerosis carry their cholesterol in association particularly with HDL. HDL are high in pre-menopause women where coronary disease is rarer than in men of the same age. HDL levels are low in coronary to

41

reduce HDL (obesity, cigarette consumption, diabetes, sedentary routine). Subjects with high LDL in familial hyperalphalipoproteinemia (HDL over 0.8 g/l) would seem to live longer. Three observations underline the purifying role of HDL in relation to tissue cholesterol. Delipidated HDL are good receivers for cholesterol cell withdrawal. HDL are also a good substrate for lecithine : cholesterol acyl transferase (LCAT) which facilitates cholesterol transfer from tissues to HDL. Finally, during slimming HDL act as a carrier for cholesterol which is released by the adipose tissue [38]. In the absence of HDL, in an alphalipoprotemia, cholesterol accumulates in the reticulo-endothelial tissue and familial hypoalphalipoprotemia is accompanied by precocious atherosclerosis [39]. A moderate alcohol intake increases HDL and gives a lower incidence of coronary mortality.

We have a long way to do before this protective mechanism is completely elucidated. The nature of the HDL fraction responsible for the cholesterol returning to the liver is still unknown. Some believe that only 5 % of HDL have this effect [40]. Moreover HDL increase is not beneficial in every case, nor is its decrease always harmful. Thus we can see that some pesticides, while increasing HDL, cannot be considered desirable [41], some cases of hypoalphalipoprotemia are not accompanied by accelerated atherosclerosis, (Apo AI-Milano [42], lipoprotein lipase deficiency), probucol lowers HDL and yet remains anti-atherogenous [43, 44] and myocardial infarction can occur in certain cases of spontaneous [45] or estrogen-induced [46] hyper-alphalipoproteinemia.

LDL/HDL ratios

The distinction between lipoproteins which carry cholesterol to the tissues, (LDL) and lipoproteins which favor its withdrawal (HDL) has led us to use the LDL/HDL ratio as an atherogenicity index [34, 47]. The terms "bad cholesterol" for LDL cholesterol and "good cholesterol" for the HDL variety, used more or less knowledgeably, have become part of household language.

The predictive value of this correlation for coronary risk has been shown to be more discriminating than that of each of its elements taken alone [34, 47, 48]. For the use of this ratio to be valid, the measurement of the HDL-cholesterol, as the denominator, must be accurate which is not always the case [49]. The slightest error can transfer a subject from one risk category to another, resulting in misinterpretation.

The value of this "atherogenicity index" has been confirmed by the large number of studies which have linked coronary risk improvement, or the degree of atheroma regression, to a decrease in the LDL/HDL ratio [23, 27, 28, 31, 50]. Preventive and regression studies [23, 31] whose results combine an increase in HDL-cholesterol with a reduction in LDL-cholesterol have been very encouraging. New interest has been generated for medicines which can have a beneficial effect on this ratio such as niacine, statines and certain fibrates.

Apolipoproteins and the metabolic destiny of lipoproteins

As knowledge progressed attention was increasingly   drawn to apolipoproteins (apo) as coronary risk mediators [51-53]. These surface proteins preside over the metabolic destiny of lipoproteins through their interaction with cell receptors, their role as enzyme activators or inhibitors and their contribution to the structure of lipoprotein particles.

Global plasma apolipoprotein B [54-56] and LDL apo B [57, 58] are as good as, if not better than, LDL cholesterol as coronary risk indicators. Conversely the protective role of HDL has been attributed to apo AI [58] and its predictive value has been considered by some as higher than that of HDL [59]. This idea has been lent weight by the discovery that the absence of apo AI [60] or a deficiency of apo AI-CIII [61] is associated with premature atheromatosis. More recently the work of the Fruchart group in Lille indicates that it is the lipoprotein particles carrying AI without apo II, the Lp AI, which are the most discriminating [62]. This notion of functionally distinct lipoprotein particles is of considerable significance in the evolution of the lipoprotein hypothesis and will be taken up in greater detail by Professor Fruchart in the course of this symposium. Some authorities have demonstrated the advantages of using an apo AI/apo B index rather than LDL/HDL [48, 53-55]. It would seem that, here again, the predictive power of this ratio is higher than that of its components taken individually. This predictive power will be proportionately greater the closer the cholesterol levels get to normal levels; this can be seen in the study described by Noma and colleagues [48].

Apolipoprotein E which is polymorphous, seems to play a modulating role on cholesterol and LDL-cholesterol levels in the population [63]. Its three forms E4, E3 and E2 differ from each other by the substitution of an amino-acid for remnants 112 and 158 of its peptide chain of 299 amino acids. They are coded at chromosome 19 by three alleles (ε2, ε3, ε4) which determine 6 common phenotypes. Apo E can interact both with the LDL receptor sites on the hepatic cell. Numerous observations lead us to believe that the polymorphous nature of apo E plays a role in the expression of atherosclerosis, by influencing LDL-cholesterol blood levels [63]. Compared to the common allele ε3, allele ε2 combines with lower levels of LDL-cholesterol (which are anti-atherogenous) but predisposes to hypertriglyceridemia (which is atherogenous) while allele ε4 combines with higher levels of LDL-cholesterol which could favor atherosclerosis. Higher ε4 allele frequency in Finns [64] whose coronary risk is greater, and in myocardial infarction subjects [65, 66] and inversely, a lower frequency of this allele among the Japanese [67] and among octogenerians [68] suggest that this allele does have an atherogenous effect. It has been shown that coronary subjects bearing allele ε4 tend to experience infarctus more precociously than carriers of allele ε2 [69]. Pedersen and Berg have recently demonstrated [70] that the impact of apo E on blood cholesterol depended on a variation of the locus of the LDL receptor, itself also located on chromosome 19. Apo E only has an effect in the absence of a PvuII restriction site for the LDL gene receptor.

Lipoprotein nature and composition influence the atherogenous potential

We are now aware the atherogenous potential of a lipoprotein is based as much as on its composition as on its blood level. Every modification of a lipoprotein, and in particular of surface lipoproteins can change its destiny. Thus VLDL (very low density lipoproteins) rich in triglycerides [71] would seem to be captured more avidly by the macrophage scavengers which act as garbage collectors, favoring the creation of spumous cells. The same is true for postlipolytic VLDL remnants which are cytotoxic for the macrophages and share this type of atherogenous potential [72]. Normal HDL would seem to act as protectors against this cytoxic effect. On the other hand the presence of abnormally composed HDL rich in triglycerides has been linked to an increased risk. In a prospective study Miettinen and colleagues [74] showed that the fatty acid composition of circulating phospholipids (measured initially) influences the risk of myocardial infarctus (5-7 years later). Saturated fatty acid content (palmitic and stearic) was higher while poly unsatured fatty acid content (linoleic, eicosapentaenoic and docosahexaenoic) was lower in coronary subjects than in their matching control subjects. This was not the case for triglyceride fatty acids and cholesterol esters. Since the greater part of the phospholipids is transported by the HDL it would seem that the HDL fatty acid composition could indirectly influence their anti-atherogenous potential. Along the same lines Naruszewicz and colleagues have shown that the LDL of subjects treated with probucol behave differently from native LDL and can be catabolised by a process which is independent of the LDL receptor. The hypothesis has been put forward that probucol, which dissolves in the non-polar LDL core, may modify apo B surface conformation and could explain its new catabolic orientation.

Lipoproteins "modified" by acetylation [76], glycosylation, or oxidation [78] prefer to direct themselves towards the macrophage in order to interact with the acetyl LDL scavenger receptor. However the accumulation of cholesterol in the intima macrophages, activated monocytes or transformed smooth muscular cells, which leads to the creation of spumous cells, constitutes a precocious atherogenesis phase. It is therefore becoming important to pay greater attention to the mechanisms which preside *in vivo* over lipoprotein modification and over their introduction into the macrophages and to obstacles which might be set up to impede these phenomena. This aspect has recently been reviewed by Steinberg and colleagues [79].

Perspectives for the future

At the same time as the lipid hypothesis developed to include lipoproteins, apolipoproteins and their molecular modifications, our therapeutic means developed, keeping up with our advancing knowledge. Modern medicines, acting on the metabolism, the composition and the conformation of lipoproteins have become veritable tools by which lipoprotein metabolism can be explored. We might quote, for example, substances which act on cholesterol synthesis [80] and on HDL metabolism [23, 81], or which protect against LDL oxidation [82]. The anti-oxidant effect of probucol which protects the Watanabe rabbit from atherosclerosis [44, 82, 83] is a breakthrough worthy of careful attention. For reasons which are still unclear it would seem that cigarette smoke carries hydrosoluble substances able to alter lipoproteins and to favor the creation of spumous cells [84]. It is interesting to note that this atherogenous potential of cigarette smoke is considerably inhibited by anti-oxidants. Thus even well-established risk factors will have to be re-appraised in the light of recent discoveries.

For a long time now we have sought to determine what might link thrombogenesis to atherogenesis; endothelium platelets have frequently been the target of research in this context. Another molecule, Lp(a) has now come to the forefront. This is a highly glucolysed polymorphous lipoprotein, present in 65 % of the population, but which has retained its mystery [85]. High Lp(a) levels (> 30 mg/dl) are associated with an increased incidence of coronary mortality [86]. Apo (a), partially masking on apo (b) the interaction site of this ligand with the LDL receptor, probably contributes to the athero-genous effect for which it is known. But the homology of the molecule with plasminogen [87] has raised the possibility of a role in thrombogenesis. This link seems to have been established recently by the demonstration that Lp (a) competes on the endothelial cell with plasminogen for its receptor and inhibits plasminogen activation this opposing plasmin synthesis [88]. Lp (a) tends to accumulate on the endothelium surface and it has been calculated that concentrations of 30 mg/dl of Lp (a) can inhibit plasmin linkage by 20 % interfering locally with fibrinolysis and creating a pro-coagulant con-dition [88].

It is not yet known whether these molecules can be oxidized and whether the product of oxidation would possess an increased atherogenous or thrombogenous potential, but there is on-going research in this area.

Research in increasingly directed towards the macrophage cell receptors which may well be at the origin of the creation of atherocytes. The recent cloning of two of these receptors [89] represents without doubt a break-through whose consequences for our understanding of the detailed workings of atherogenesis have already been outlined [90]. Several laboratories are also concentrating on the hereditary mechanisms rendering the arterial wall more or less resistant to lipoprotein aggression. Among others should be quoted the work of Paigen and colleagues [91] and of Stewart-Phillips and colleagues [92] who have sought the genetic determinants of atherosclerosis susceptibility and resistance in pure mice strains. For example strain C57BL/J6 is susceptible to diet induced atherosclerosis while strain A/J is resistant. In both cases serum cholesterol increases with the diet, but in the resistant mouse HDL cholesterol increases, while in the susceptible strain it decreases [92]. The differences are attributed to gene ATH3 on mouse chro-mosome 7 which has homologous sequences on the human chromosome 19 near the apo E site; here again lipoproteins and apolipoproteins remain at the heart of the debate.

References

1. Davignon J. Current views on the etiology and pathogenesis of atherosclerosis. *In : Hyper-tension : physiopathology and treatment.* J Genest E. Koïw and O. Küchel (eds.) McGraw-Hill, New York, 1977; pp. 961-989.

2. Davignon J, Dufour R, Cantin M. Atherosclerosis and hypertension. *In : Hypertension : physiopathology and treatment.* J Genest, O. Küchel, P. Hamet and M. Cantin (eds). McGraw-Hill, New York, 1983; pp. 810-852.

3. Benditt EP. Origins of human atherosclerotic plaques. Arch Pathol Lab Med 1988; 112 : 997-1001.

4. Schwartz CJ, Valente AJ, Kelley JL *et al.* Thrombosis and the development of atherosclerosis : Rokitanski revisited. Semin Thromb Hemost 1988; 14 : 189-195.

5. Ross R. Atherosclerosis ; a problem of the biology of arterial wall cells and their interactions with blood components. Arteriosclerosis 1981; 1 : 293-311.

6. Ross R. Pathogenesis of atherosclerosis : an update. N Engl J Med 1986; 314 : 488-500.

7. Hansson GK, Schwartz SM. Endothelial cell dysfunction without cell loss. *In : Biochemical interactions at the endothelium* Cryer A (ed). Elsevier, New York, 1983; pp. 343-361.

8. Cotran R. New roles for the endothelium in inflammation and immunity. Am J Path 1987; 129 : 407-413.

9. Koo EWY, Gotlieb AI. Endothelial stimulation of intimal cell proliferation in a porcine aortic organ culture. Am J Path 1989; 134 ; 497-503.

10. Hansson GK, Jonasson K, Seifert PS *et al.* Immune mechanisms in atherosclerosis. Arteriosclerosis 1989; 9 : 567-578.

11. Hopkins PN, Williams RR. A survey of 246 suggested coronary risk factors. Atherosclerosis 1981; 40 : 1-51.

12. Astrupp P, Kjeldsen K. Carbon monoxide, smoking and atherosclerosis. Med Clin North Am 1974; 58 : 323.

13. Texon M. Mechanical factors involved in atherosclerosis. *In : Atherosclerotic vascular disease : a Hahnemann Symposium.* AN Brest, JH Moyer (eds). Appleton-Century-Crofts, New York, 1967; p. 23.

14. Bell FB, Somer JB, Craig IH *et al.* Patterns of aortic Evans blue uptake *in vivo* and *in vitro.* Atherosclerosis 1972; 16 : 69-375.

15. Haimovici H, Mater N. Role of arterial tissue susceptibility in experimental canine atherosclerosis. J Atheroscler Res 1966; 6 : 62.

16. Glagov S. Mechanical stresses on vessels and the non-uniform distribution of atherosclerosis. Med Clin North Am 1973; 57 : 63.

17. Clarkson TM, Bond MG, Bullock BC *et al.* A study of atherosclerosis regression in Macaca mulatta. IV- Changes in coronary arteries from animals with atherosclerosis induced for 19 months and then regressed for 24 or 48 months at plasma cholesterol concentrations of 300 or 200 mg/dl. Exp Mol Pathol 1981; 34 : 345-368.

18. Wissler RW, Vesselinovitch d. Combined effects of cholestyramine and probucol on regression of atherosclerosis in rhesus monkey aortas. Appl Pathol 1983; 1 : 89-96.

19. Moore S. Endothelial injury and atherosclerosis. Exper Mol Pathol 1979; 31 : 182-190.

20. Thomas Wa, Florentin RA, Nam SC *et al.* Plasma lipids and experimental atherosclerosis. *In : Athero-sclerosis : Proceedings of the Second International Symposium.* RJ Jones (ed). Springer-Verlag, New York, 1970; pp. 414-426.

21. Hjermann I, Velvebyre K, Holme I *et al.* Effect of diet and smoking intervention on the incidence of coronary heart disease. Report from the Oslo Study Group of a randomized trial in healthy man. Lancet 1981; 2 : 1303-1313.

22. Lipid Research Clinic Program. The Lipid Research Clinics Coronary Primary Prevention Trial Results. J Amer Med Assoc 1984; 251 : 351-374.

23. Frick MH, Elo O, Haapa K *et al.* Helsinki Heart Study : primary-prevention trial with gemfibrozil in middle-aged men with dyslipidemia. Safety of treatment, changes in risk factors and incidence of coronary heart disease. New Engl J Med 1987; 317 : 1237-1245.

24. Ost Cr, Stenson S. Regression of peripheral atherosclerosis during therapy with high doses of nicotinic acid. Scand J Clin Lab Invest 1967; (Supp) 99 : 241-245.

25. Basta LL, Williams C, Kioschos JM *et al*. Regression of atherosclerotic stenosing lesions of the renal arteries and spontaneous cure of systemic hypertension through control of hyperlipidemia. Am J Med 1976; 61 : 420-422.

26. Barndt R Jr, Blankenhorn DH, Crawford DW *et al*. Regression and progression of early femoral atherosclerosis in treated hyperlipoproteinemic patients. Ann Intern Med 1977; 86 : 139-146.

27. Duffied RGM, Miller NE, Brunt JNH *et al*. Treatment of hyperlipidaemia retards progression of symptomatic femoral atherosclerosis – A randomized controlled trial. Lancet 1983; 2 : 639-642.

28. Nikkila EA, Viikinkoski P, Valle M *et al*. Prevention of progression of coronary atherosclerosis by treatment of hyperlipidaemia : a seven year prospective angiographic study. Br Med J 1984; 289 : 220-223.

29. Brensike JF, Levy RI, Kelsey SF *et al*. Effects of therapy with cholestyramine on progression of coronary arteriosclerosis : results of the NHLBI type II coronary intervention study. Circulation 1984; 69 : 313-324.

30. Kuo PT, Haysase K, Kostis JB *et al*. Use of combined diet and colestipol in long-term (7-7.5 years) treatment of patients with type II hyperlipoproteinemia. Circulation 1979; 59 : 199-211.

31. Blankenhorn DH, Nessim SA, Johnson RL *et al*. Beneficial effects of combined colestipol-niacin thepary on coronary atherosclerosis and coronary venous bypass grafts. JAMA 1987; 257 : 3233-3240.

32. Davignon J, Lussier-Cacan S, Ortin-George M *et al*. Plasma lipids and lipoprotein patterns in angiographically graded atherosclerosis of the legs and in coronary heart disease. Can Med Assoc J 1977; 116 : 1245-1250.

33. Keys A (ed). Coronary heart disease in seven countries. Circulation 1970; 41 (Supp 1) : I-1-I-211.

34. Kannel WB, Castelli WP, Gordon T. Cholesterol in the prediction of atherosclerotic disease – New perspectives based on the Framingham study. Ann Intern Med 1979; 90 : 85-91.

35. Watanabe Y. Serial inbreeding of rabbits with hereditary hyperlipidemia (WHHL-rabbit) – Incidence and development of atherosclerosis and xanthoma. Atherosclerosis 1980; 36 : 261-268.

36. Newman WP, Freedman DS, Voors AW *et al*. Relation of serum lipoprotein levels and systolic blood pressure to early atherosclerosis. The Bogalusa Heart Study. New Engl J Med 1986; 314 : 138-144.

37. Miller GJ, Miller NE. Plasma high density lipoprotein concentration and development of ischaemic heart disease. Lancet 1975; 1 : 16-19.

38. Nnestel PJ, Miller NE. Mobilization of adipose tissue cholesterol in high density lipoprotein during weight reduction in man. *In : High density lipoproteins and atherosclerosis*. AM Gotto Jr, NE Miller, MF Oliver (eds). Elsevier/North Holland, 1978; pp. 51-54.

39. Vergagni C, Bettale G. Familial hypoalphalipoproteinemia. Clin Chim Acta 1981; 114 : 45-62.

40. Fielding CJ, Fielding PE. Cholesterol transport between cells and body fluids. Role of plasma lipoproteins and the plasma cholesterol esterification system. Med Clin N Amer 1982; 66 : 363-373.

41. Carlson LA, Kolomodin-Hedman B. Hyperalphalipoproteinemia in men exposed to chlorinated hydrocarbon pesticides. Acta Med Scand 972; 192 : 29.

42. Franceschini G, Sirtrori CR, Capurso A *et al.* AI Milano apoprotein. Decreased high density lipoprotein cholesterol levels with significant lipoprotein modifications and without clinical atherosclerosis in an Italian family. J Clin Invest 1980; 66 : 892-900.

43. Davignon J, Bouthillier D. Probucol and familial hypercholesterolemia. Can Med Asso J 1982; 126 : 1024-1025.

44. Kita T, Nagano Y, Yokode M *et al.* Probucol prevents the progression of atherosclerosis in the Watanabe heritable hyperlipidemic rabbit, an animal model for familial hypercholesterolemia. Proc Natl Acad Sci (USA) 1987; 84 : 5928-5931.

45. Rotsztain A. Risk factors and HDL. Circulation 1978; 57 : 1032.

46. Stamler J. Dietary and serum lipids in the multifactorial etiology of atherosclerosis. Arch Surg 1978; 113 ; 21-25.

47. Castelli WP. HDL in assessing risk of CHD. Metab Therap 1977; 6 : 1-3.

48. Noma A, Yokosura T, Kitamura K. Plasma lipids and apolipoproteins are discriminators for presence and severity of angiographically defined coronary artery disease. Atherosclerosis 1983; 49 : 1-7.

49. Warnick GR, Albers JJ, Leary ET. HDL cholesterol : Results of interlaboratory proficiency tests. Clin Chem 1980; 26 : 169-170.

50. Arntzenius AC, Kromhout D, Barth JD *et al.* Diet, lipoproteins and the progression of coronary atherosclerosis. The leiden Intervention Trial. N Engl J Med 1985; 312 : 805-811.

51. Thompson G. Apoproteins : determinants of lipoprotein metabolism and indices of coronary risk. Br Heart J 1984; 51 : 585-588.

52. Mahley RW, Innerarity TL, Rall Sc Jr *et al.* Plasma lipoproteins : apolipoproteins structure and function. J Lipid Res 1985; 25 : 1277-1294.

53. Alaupovic P, McConathy WJ, Fesmire J *et al.* Profiles of apolipoproteins and apolipoprotein B-containing lipoprotein particles in dyslipoproteinema. Clin Chem 1988; 34 : B13-B27.

54. Avogaro P, Bittolo Bon G, Cazzolato G *et al.* Are apolipoproteins better discriminators than lipids for atherosclerosis ? Lancet 1979; 1 : 901-903.

55. Fruchart JC, Parra H, Cachera C *et al.* Lipoproteins, apolipoproteins and coronary artery disease. Ric Clin Lab 1982; 12 : 101-106.

56. Kladetsky RG, Assmann G, Walgenbach S *et al.* Lipoprotein and apoprotein values in coronary angiography patients. Artery 1980; 7 : 191-205.

57. Brunzell JD, Sniderman AD, Albers JJ *et al.* Apoproteins B and A-I and coronary artery disease in humans. Artheriosclerosis 1984; 4 : 79-83.

58. Sniderman AD. Polippoprotein B and apolipoprotein AI as predictors of coronary artery disease. Can J Cardiol 1988; 4 : 24A-30A.

59. Maciejko JJ, Holmes DR, Kottke B *et al.* Apoprotein AI as a marker of angiographically assessed coronary-artery disease. New Engl J Med 1983; 309 : 385-389.

60. Norum RA, Lakier JB, Goldstein S *et al.* Familial deficiency of apolipoprotein AI and CIII and precocious coronary-artery disease. New Engl J Med 1982; 306 : 1513-1519.

61. Schaefer EJ, Heaton WH, Wetzel MG *et al.* Plasma apolipoprotein A-I absence associated with a marked reduction of high density lipoproteins and premature coronary heart disease. Arteriosclerosis 1982; 2 : 16-26.

62. Puchois P, Kandoussi A, Fievet P *et al.* Apolipoprotein AI-containing lipoproteins in coronary artery disease. Atherosclerosis 1987; 68 : 35-40.

63. Davignon J, Gregg RE, Sing CF. Apolipoprotein E polymorphism and atherosclerosis. Arteriosclerosis 1988; 8 : 1-21.

64. Ehnholm C, Lukka M, Kuusi T *et al*. Apolipoprotein E polymorphism in the Finnish population : gene frequencies and relation to lipoprotein concentrations. J Lipid Res 1986; 27 : 227-235.

65. Kuusi T, Nieminen MS, Enholm C *et al*. Apoprotein E polymorphism and coronary artery disease – Increased prevalence of apolipoprotein E4 in angiographically verified coronary patients. Arteriosclerosis 1989; 9 : 237-241.

66. Cumming AM, Robertson F. Polymorphism at the apo E locus in relation to risk of coronary disease. Clin Genet 1984; 25 : 310.

67. Yamamura T, Yamamoto A, Hiramori K *et al*. A new isoform of apolipoprotein B – apo E-5 – associated with hyperlipidemia and atherosclerosis. Atherosclerosis 1984; 50 : 159-172.

68. Davignon J, Bouthillier D, Nestruck AC *et al*. Apolipoprotein E polymorphism and atherosclerosis : Insight from a study in octogenarians. Trans Amer Clin Climatol Assoc 1987; 99 : 100-110.

69. Lenzen HJ, Assmann G, Buchwalsky R *et al*. Association of apolipoprotein E polymorphism, low density lipoprotein cholesterol, and coronary artery disease. Clin Chem 1986; 32 : 778-781.

70. Pedersen JR, Berg K. Interaction between low density lipoprotein receptor (LDLR) and apolipoprotein E (apoE) alleles contributes to normal variation in lipid level. Clin Gene 1989 ; 35; 331-337.

71. Gianturco SH, Gotto AM Jr, Bradley WA. Hypertriglyceridemia : lipoprotein receptors and atherosclerosis. Adv Exper Med 1985: 183; 47-71.

72. Chung BH, Segrest JP, Smith K *et al*. Lipolytic surface remnants of triglyceride-rich lipoproteins are cytotoxic to macrophages but not in the presence of high density lipoprotein – A possible mechanism of atherogenesis ? J Clin Invest 1989; 83 : 1363-1374.

73. Kakis G, Feather T, Little JA. Plasma high density lipoprotein triglyceride as a risk factor for ischemic vascular disease : A prospective study. Artheriosclerosis 1983; 3 : 480a.

74. Miettinen TA, Naukkarinen V, Huttunen JK *et al*. Fatty-acid composition of serum lipids predicts myocardial infarction. Brit Med J 1982; 285 : 993-996.

75. Naruszewicz M, Carew TE, Pitman RC *et al*. A novel mechanism by which probucol lowers low density lipoprotein levels demonstrated in the LDL receptor-deficient rabbit. J Lipid Res 1984; 25 : 1206-1213.

76. Golstein JL, Ho YK, Basu SK *et al*. Binding site on macrophages that mediates uptake and degradation of acetylated low density lipoprotein, producing massive cholesterol deposition. Proc Natl Acad Sci (USA) 1979; 76 : 333-337.

77. Witztum JL, Mahoney EM, Branks MJ *et al*. Nonenzymatic glycosylation of low density lipoproteins alters its biological activity Diabetes 1981; 31 : 283-291.

78. Parthasarathy S, Fong L, Otero D *et al*. Recognition of solubilized apoproteins from delipidated, oxidized low density lipoprotein (LDL) by the acetyl-LDL receptor. Proc Nat Acad Sci (USA) 1987; 84 : 537-540.

79. Steinberg D, Parthasarathy S, Carew TE *et al*. Beyond cholesterol. Modification of low-density lipoprotein that increase its atherogenicity. N Engl J Med 1989; 320 : 915-924.

80. Endo A, Kuroda M, Tanzawa K. Competitive inhibition of 3-hydroxy-3-methylglutaryl coenzyme A reductase by ML-236A and ML-236B fungal metabolites, having hypocholesterolemic activity. FEBS Lett 1976; 72 : 323-326.

81. Carlson LA, Oro L. Effect of treatment with nicotinic acid for one month on serum lipids in patients with different types of hyperlipidemia. Atherosclerosis 1973; 18 : 1-9.

82. Steinberg D. Studies on the mechanism of action of probucol. Am J Cardiol 1986; 57 : 16H-21H.

83. Carew TE, Schwenke DC, Steinberg D. Antiatherogenic effect of probucol unrelated to its hypocholesterolemic effect : evidence that antioxidants *in vivo* can selectively inhibit low density lipoprotein degradation in macrophage-rich fatty streaks and slow the progression of atherosclerosis in the Watanabe heritable hyperlipidemic rabbit. Proc Natl Acad Sci (USA) 1987; 84 : 7725-7729.

84. Yokode M, Kita T, Arai H *et al*. Cholesterol ester accumulation in macrophages incubated with low density lipoprotein pretreated with cigarette smoke extract. Proc Natl Acad Sci (USA) 1988; 85 : 2344-2348.

85. Utermann G. The Mysteries of lipoprotein(a). Science 1989; 246 : 904-910.

86. Rhoads GG, Dhalen G, Berg K *et al*. Lp(a) lipoprotein as a risk factor for myocardial infarction. JAMA 1986; 256 : 2540-2544.

87. Eaton DL, Fless GM, Kohr WJ *et al*. Partial amino acid sequence of apolipoprotein(a) shows that it is homologous to plasminogen. Proc Natl Acad Sci (USA) 1987; 84 : 3224-3228.

88. Scott J. Thrombogenesis linked to thrombogenesis at last ? Nature 1989; 341 : 22-23.

89. Rohrer L, Freeman M, Kodama T *et al*. Coiled-coil fibrous domains mediate ligand binding by macrophage scavenger receptor II. Nature 1989; 343 : 570-572.

90. Brown MS, Goldstein JL. Scavenging for receptors. Nature 1989; 343 : 508-509.

91. Paigen B, Mitchell D, Rueu K *et al*. Ath-1, a gene determining atherosclerosis susceptibility and high density lipoprotein levels in mice. Proc Natl Acad Sci (USA) 1987; 84 : 3763-3767.

92. Stewart-Phillips JL, Lough J, Skamene E. Genetically determined susceptibility and resistance to diet-induced atherosclerosis in inbred strains of mice. J Lab Clin Med 1988; 112 : 36-42.

Fish oil and blood-vessel wall interactions. Eds P.M. Vanhoutte, Ph. Douste-Blazy.
John Libbey Eurotext, Paris © 1991, pp.53 -62.

5

The effect of polyunsaturated Ω-3 fatty acids on blood lipids and lipoprotein metabolism

B. Jacotot

Research unit, Dislipidemia and Atherosclerosis, INSERM U32, Henri-Mondor Hospital, 94010 Creteil Cedex, France.

Abstract

Several epidemiological studies support the hypothese of a hypolipidemia effect of the consumption of fish oils rich in n-3 acid. The decrease in cardio-vascular disease observed in some studies could be, at least partly, a consequence of this hypolipidemia effect. Long chain n-3 fatty acid (eicosapentanoic and docosapentanoic) have essentially a hypo-triglyceridemia effect on blood lipids, clearer in patients with type IV or V hypertri-glyceridemia, and this effect is dose-related. It is above all explained by the action of fish oil on VLDL metabolism, through the inhibition of certain enzymes active in the synthesis of fatty acids and triglycerides, with the creation and secretion of smaller and denser VLDL. The effect on chylomicrons is less clear, and the process as yet not well known. Fish oils do not appear to act directly on LDL and HDL metabolism, but work will be necessary to elucidate this point and to assess the role of these oils on certain lipoprotein characteristics which may influence their atherogenicity.

Since the first observation by Bang and Dyerberg [1] pointing out a corre-lation between a high fatty fish and marine mammal food intake, and a low myocardial infarction rate among Eskimos, an increasing amount of work has been devoted to attempting to explain the processes and the clinical interest of the very long chain Ω-3 family of fatty acid. The favourable cardio-vascular effects observed [2] were in fact attributed and the role of

53

Table I. The main families of polyunsaturated fatty acids and their origins.

Initial fatty acid	Main metabolites	Origins
Ω3α-Linoleic (essential) 18:3	Eicosapentaenoic 20:5	18:3 certain vegetable oils
	Docosahexaenoic 22:6	20:5 & 22:6 fish and sea mammals
Ω6 Linoleic (essential)	Arachidonic 20:4	18:2 vegetable oils 20:4 meat, eggs
Ω9 Oleic 18:1	Eicosatrienoic 20:3	18:1 animal and vegetable fats

these fatty acids found in large quantities in the oils extracted from these marine creatures.

There has been a build-up of epidemiological data containing nevertheless some contradictions : thus a close inverse correlation between the consumption of fats and coronary death has been observed among Japanese fishermen and farmers [3, 4]; in a study undertaken in Holland, Kromhout *et al.* [5] demonstrated (by means of a 20 years follow-up) that coronary death among persons consuming 30 g or more of fish per day were half as many as those of persons with no fish intake. This correlation confirmed by others [6, 7] has not however been found to be invariable in every case [8, 9]. In a study on secondary prevention of myocardial infarction, Burr *et al.* have shown that an increase in fish intake resulted in a significant decrease in secondary death but not in infarction recurrence [10]. In this study however the rapidity of the diet effect on mortality leads us to think that the beneficial action was due above all to a favorable effect on hemostasis and coagulation mechanisms and not to an effect on blood lipids.

The interpretation of the results of epidemiological cardio-vascular studies is difficult here since the events observed (mainly myocardial infarction and coronary death) are due to several pathological processes : atherosclerosis, thrombosis, rhythmic disorders; these are integrated and generally inter-dependent but the factors triggering them are not always the same. The components of fish oils act to prevent coronary accidents through hemostasis and clot formation, through effects on lipids and lipoproteins and probably also through an effect on arterial blood pressure and cardial rhythm.

The flesh of fatty fish in particular of the cold sea varieties (salmon, herring, cod) and that of marine mammals is rich in polyunsaturated fatty acids, unlike that of land based mammals whose flesh tends to be rich in saturated fatty acids. In fact the two most commonly found polyunsaturated fatty acids in marine creatures are eicosapentaenoic acid (EPA) and docosahexaenoic acid (DHA), both belonging to the Ω-3 family (led by alpha-linoleic acid).

When a person's diet contains large quantities of these fatty acids they partially replace in the organism another polyunsaturated fatty acid, arachidonic acid, a product of the Ω-6 family (that linoleic acid).

Arachidonic acid is the sustrate from which major compounds such as certain prostaglandins and leucotriens are formed. Bearing in mind the significant role played by the metabolites of arachidonic acid in the process of platelet aggregation and cellular multiplication, it is easier to understand the consequences which might result from a modification in the equilibrium existing between these different fatty acids.

The action of Ω-3 fatty acids on blood lipids has been well known for some time; it affects above all triglycerides and very low density lipoproteins (VLDL). However the way in which these fatty acids bring about their effect on lipids and lipoproteins has not yet been clearly elucidated and published results have frequently been contradictory [11].

Lipoproteins and lipoprotein receptors

Blood lipids, cholesterol, triglycerides and phospholipids are carried in the form of lipoproteins. These are spherical aggregates with an apolar core made up of phospholipids free cholesterol and specific proteins known as apoproteins. The physiology of lipoproteins which is now wellknown has enabled us to define 3 main categories :

- those responsible for carrying lipids, originating in the intestine, to the liver and which are characterized by the presence of apo B48; these are the chylomicrons and their remnants after degradation;

- those which carry lipids originating in the liver and send them to different tissues (characterized by the presence of apo B 100); theses are the low density lipoproteins (VLDL and LDL); the transformation of VLDL into LDL takes the form of a metabolic "cascade effect" occuring in the plasma

- finally those which bring cholesterol to its excretion sites, the liver and bile vessels (characterized by two predominating apoproteins : apo A-I and apo A-II); these are the high density lipoproteins (HDL).

For each of these lipoprotein categories there is intense metabolic activity, resulting in the determination of the plasma concentration of the different particles and consequently establishing the blood levels of the lipids which they contain (cholesterol, triglycerides and phospholipids). The main stages of lipoprotein metabolism are : their secretion in the blood; alterations to their composition while in the blood stream : degradation through the effect of lipolytic enzymes, exchanges with other categories of lipoproteins, with the net result of losses gains in lipids and proteins; their disappearance from the blood through diverse channels, of which the most significant are those in which specific receptors act as mediators. Apart from these "normal" lipoproteins there are also other specific lipoproteins usually present in very low quantities, but which can play an important physio-pathological role, especially when their concentration increases in the blood or in other tissues, these are Lp(a) and "modified" LDL. Similar to LDL, LP(a) is characterized by a protein copula combining apoB and apo (a). Lp(a) serum concentration bears a high positive correlation to atheromatous illness and a high concentration represents a risk, independently of myocardial infarction. Serum concentration is genetically determined and seems not to be influenced by dietary or medicinal factors.

Modified LDL are considered as responsible for one of the key stages in atherosclerosis pathogenesis : the appearance of spumous cells in the arterial intima. Various LDL modifications are known (acetylation, malonaldehyde treatment, oxidation, combination with polysaccharides or antibodies). Modified LDL have this in particular that they do not bind to specific apo B receptors, but with macrophage receptors. This is essentially a tissue process and has been demonstrated in the arterial wall, as reponsible for macrophage immobilisation and transformation into spumous cells.

Various sorts of receptors play an essential role in lipoprotein catabolism. The first to be identified, by Goldstein and Brown [12] were the LDL receptors. LDL endocytosis is the consequence of LDL apo B100 binding with a specific site known as the apo B, E receptor (since it also recognizes another apoprotein apo E). LDL is then enveloped by an endocytosis vesicle, then downgraded by lyposomial enzymes. This mechanism plays an essential role in the regulation of intra-cellular cholesterol. Although they are present on cell membranes in all tissues, apo B, E receptors are to be found mainly in the area of the liver. The structure and characteristics of the LDL receptor are now well-known as is the pathology of the interactions between apo B, E and lipoproteins.

The apo E receptor is present only in the area of the liver; it recognizes lipoproteins containing apo E, that is to say above all remnants of chylomicrons and VLDL. Unlike apo B, E receptors, which age or vary according to physiological or nutritional factors, the activity of apo E receptors seems to be relatively stable and independent of physiological conditions.

HDL receptors are much less well-known. Specific apo A-I receptors have been identified in different organs (liver, intestine, suprarenal). Binding would seem not to be followed by envelopment but to be accompanied by a cellular cholesterol transfer to HDL, the latter being subsequently released. This process is an important step in the cholesterol "return journey".

Finally, as already mentioned, there are macrophage receptors, susceptible of binding pathological lipoproteins and which could play a role in the initial stages of the atherosclerosis lesion.

Effect of Ω-3 fatty acids on plasma lipids

A recent review by Harris [11] based on 45 publications was devoted to this subject. The oils were most frequently Ω-3 fatty acid* or oils from the flesh of different fish (mackerel, herring, pogy) and in some cases cod liver oil (*Figure 1*).

We must first of all stress the high level of heterogeneity in the procedures adopted, especially in the daily doses of fish extract employed. These doses ranged from 4 g/day to 100 g/day in some studies. The main effect observed concerned the triglyceride (TG) concentration. This decreased regularly with a clear dose-effect both in normolipidic and in hyperlipidemia subjects. Thus, in the case of normolipidemic subjects, the TG decrease varie from 1 to 30 % with doses of from 4 to 10 g/day, from 12 to 48 % with doses of from

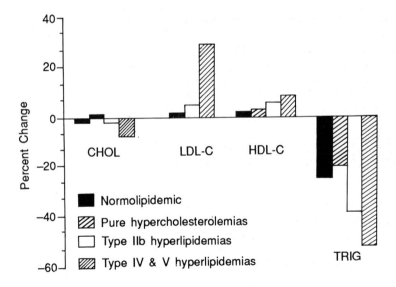

Figure 1. Mean percentage modification of blood lipids observed in 45 publications, based on Harris [11].

(*) Maxepa ®.

10 to 20 g/day, and from 40 to 60 % with doses of from 20 to 100 g/day. In the case of type IIB hyperlipidemia subjects (mixed hyperlipidemia) the TG decrease was from 17 to 38 % for a dose of from 5 to 12 g/day, from 40 to 50 % for from 18 to 20 g/day and from 40 to 65 % for from 75 to 112 g/day. Finally in type IV or V hyperlipidemia cases the TG decrease was from 26 to 61 % for doses 10 to 20 g/day, from 55 to 70 % for 50 g/day and from 66 to 81 % for 75 g/day.

The effect on LDL cholesterol is irregular and in any case weak in normolipidemic subjects. In type IIb subjects a moderate (max 16 %) increase was noted, except for one publication (decrease of 12 % with a dose of 20 g/day). For types IV and V, an increase of from 18 to 63 % was observed in the 7 studies where this parameter was measured. HDL cholesterol modification was inconsistent, and varied with the study both for normolipidemic and for type IIb subjects. In types IV and V an increase for this parameter, in the region of 10 to 20 %, was observed, independently of the dose. These results are summarized in *Figure 1* based on Harris [11].

Effect on plasma apoproteins

Results obtained for apoB concentration are parallel to those for LDL cholesterol.

As far as apo A-1 are concerned a slight decrease was noted in normolipidemic subjects, while there was practically no effect for types IIb and IV. Apoprotein E could be diminished for types V.

The effect on Lp(a) is not yet well known. In a recent work [13] on coronary and hypertension subjects undergoing regular physical training, an average decrease of 15 % in Lp(a) was noted for subjects receiving Ω-3 fatty acid for 4 weeks, compared to others receiving a vegetal polyunsaturated oil.

Effect on lipoprotein metabolism

VLDL metabolism *(Figures 2 and 3)*

It is here that the action of Ω-3 fatty acid can be seen most clearly. The main targets are the hepatic synthesis of fatty acids and of triglycerides, and the synthesis and excretion of VLDL.

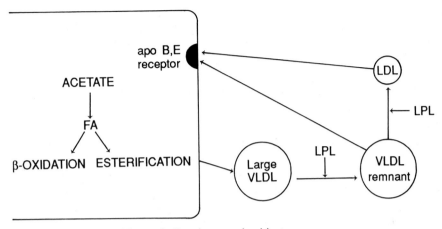

Figure 2. Diagram : LLDL metabolism in normal subject.

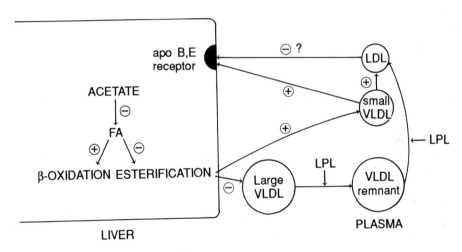

Figure 3. Diagram : VLDL metabolism and modifications observed during treatment by Ω-3 fatty acid, based on Harris [11].

Fatty acid synthesis is decreased by the inhibition of certain enzymes, particularly acetyl Co-A carboxylase. In addition the $\Delta 6$ and $\Delta 9$ desaturases are also eliminated. On the other hand there does seem to be an increase in beta-oxidation which contributes to a decrease in the fatty acid concentration.

The esterification of fatty acids leading to triglyceride synthesis, is decreased, in particular through the inhibition of diacylglycerol-acyl-transferase.

59

VLDL synthesis is decreased as a result of the decrease in hepatic triglycerides and a fewer secretion by hepatocyte of large VLDL rich in TG; there is also a secretion of small VLDL which are denser due to the decrease in TG whose catabolism is accelerated (faster transformation into LDL and improved capture by apoB, E receptors).

On the other hand fish oils have an effect on lipoprotein-lipase nor on hepatic triglyceride-lipase.

Chylomicron metabolism

The effect of fish oils is less clear. There is probably a decrease in the intestinal synthesis of chylomicrons, not so much through the effect of intestinal absorption of fatty acid, but rather through a decrease in fatty acids and TG synthesis in the enterocytes. Fish oils also cause an increase in chylomicron catabolism; this is not due to stimulation of plasma or hepatic lipotrotein-lipases; moreover the presence of fatty acids in Ω-3 in the chylomicrons does not affect their clearance. One hypothesis is that lipoprotein-lipase may be more competitive in its action on chylomicrons given the decrease in VLDL.

LDL metabolism

Plasma LDL concentration appears to increase mainly because of an accelerated transformation of small dense VLDL into LDL. Moreover the catabolism of LDL appears to decrease, not as a result of the action of fish oils on apoB, E receptors, but through a competition effect on small VLDL whose binding on to the receptors is enhanced.

Table II. Essential fatty acid : metabolism

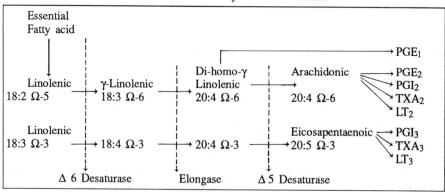

Table III. Main characteristics of different human plasma lipoproteins

Lipoproteins	Density (g/ml)	Diameter (mm)	Mobility (in agarose gel)	% lipids	% proteins	Main lipids % of total	Main apoproteins
Chylomicrons	< 0.95	100-500	origin	98	2	Triglycerides 90 %	A,B,C
VLDL	0.95-1.006	30-100	pre.β	92	8	Triglycerides 60 % Phospholipids 15 % Cholesterol 45 %	B,C,E
IDL	1.006-1.019	25-30	β			Triglycerides 35 % Phospholipids 15 % Cholesterol 45 %	B,C,E
LDL	1.019-1.063	20-35	β	75	25	Phospholipids 30 % Cholesterol 60 %	B
HDL	1.063-1.21	10		45-60	40-55	Phospholipids 40 % Cholesterol 40 %	A,C,E

Another aspect of LDL metabolism is their atherogenicity. The atherogenous nature of LDL can notably be modified by the degree of lipoprotein fluidity. It is well known that LDL and HDL fluidity can be influenced by certain alimentary lipids [14]. Little information is available on the effect of fish oil on this parameter. Work must also be done to assess LDL sensitivity to oxidizing agents in subjects receiving fish oil. We know in fact that the more recent theories on atherosclerosis bring into play modified, notably oxidized, LDL, in the creation of spumous arterial wall cells.

HDL metabolism

No study is currently available on the effect of fish oil on HDL metabolism, in particular on receptor of cell cholesterol by HDL and other lipoproteins, their interaction with membrane receptors, exchanges between HDL and other lipoproteins, all of which are important processes in the cholesterol return journey.

Conclusion

Treatment by fish oils brings an interesting contribution to the reduction of plasma triglycerides in hyperlipidemia associated with increased VLDL i.e. types IV and V. This effect is particularly significant in the role it plays in decreasing the risk of acute pancreatitis high hypertriglyceridemia. There remains nevertheless a degree of uncertainty as far as the prevention of coronary disease is concerned insofar as the atherogenous nature of type IV hypertriglyceridemia appears to be relatively insignificant, and as long as we are short on data concerning the effects of fish oils on LDL and HDL. More work will be necessary on the points.

Finally the interest of fish oils for secondary hyperlipidemia (diabetes, chronic renal failure, organ transplants) may have considerable potential and could justify further investigation.

References

1. Bang HO, Dyerberg J. Plasma lipids and lipoproteins in Greenlandic west coast Eskimos. Am J Clin Nutr 1972; 192 : 85-94.

2. Dyerberg J, Bang HO Stoffersen HO *et al.* Eicosapentaenoic acid and prevention of thrombosis and atherosclerosis. Lancet 1978; 2 : 117-9.

3. Kagawa Y, Nishizawa M, Suzuki M *et al.* Eicosapolyenoic acid of serum lipids of Japanese islanders with low incidence of cardiovascular diseases. J Nutr Sci Vitaminol (Tokyo) 1982; 28 : 441-53.

4. Hirai A, Hamaza KL, Terano T *et al.* Eicosapentaenoic acid and platelet function in Japanese. Lecet 1980; 2 : 1132-3.

5. Kromhout D, Bosschiete EB, De Lezenne Coulander C. The inverse relation between fish consumption and 20-year mortality from coronary heart disease. New Engl J Med 1985; 312 : 1205-9.

6. Shekelle RB, Paul O, Shryock AM *et al.* Fish consumption and mortality from coronary heart disease. New Engl J Med 1985; 313 : 820.

7. Norell SE, Ahlbolm A, Feychting M *et al.* Fish consumption and mortality from coronary heart disease. Brit Med J 1986; 293 : 426.

8. Vollset SE, Heuch I, Bjelke E. Fish consumption and mortality from coronary heart disease. New Engl J Med 1985; 313 : 821.

9. Curb JD, Reed DM. Fish consumption and mortality from coronary heart disease. New Engl J Med 1985; 313 : 821.

10. Burr ML, Gilbert JF, Holliday RM *et al.* Effect of changes in fat, fish, and fibre intakes on death and myocardial reinfarction : diet and reinfarction trial (DART). Lancet 1989; 2 : 757-761.

11. Harris WS. Fish oils and plasma lipid and lipoprotein metabolism in humans : in critical review. J Lipid Res 1989; 30 : 785-802.

12. Goldstein JL, Brown MS. Binding and degradation of low density lipoproteins by cultured human fibroblasts : Comparison of cells from a normal subject and from patient with homozygous familial hypercholesterolemia. J. Biol Chem 1974; 249 ; 5153.

13. Herrmann W, Biermann J, Lindhofer HG *et al.* Beeinflussung des atherogenen riskofactors Lp(a) durch supplementäre Fischölaufnahme bei Patienten mit moderaten physischen training. Med Klin 1989; 84 : 429.

14. Sola-Alberich R, Baudet MF, Motta C *et al.* Effects of dietary fats on the fluidity of human high density lipoprotein : influence of the overall composition and phospholipid fatty acids. Biochim Biophy Acta 1990; in press.

15. Steinberg D, Parthasarathy S, Carew TE *et al.* Beyond cholesterol : modifications of low-density lipoprotein that increase its atherogenicity. New Engl J Med 1989; 320 : 915-924.

Fish oil and blood-vessel wall interactions. Eds P.M. Vanhoutte, Ph. Douste-Blazy.
John Libbey Eurotext, Paris © 1991, pp. 63-67.

6

Interaction between Ω-3 fatty acid and platelet phospholipids

M. Lagarde, M. Groset, M. Hajarine

INSERM U205, Chimie biologique INSA, Bât. 406, 69621 Villeurbanne, France.

Abstract

Ω-3 fatty acids, ingested from fish fat, have been recognized as potential inhibitors of some processes involved in atherogenesis and thrombogenesis. Among these, platelet hyperactivity may be efficiently reduced by the two main Ω-3 fatty acids of fish oil, namely eicosapentaenoic (Epa, 20:5 Ω-3) and docosahexaenoic (DHA, 22:6 Ω-3) acids, both *in vivo* and *in vitro*. Most of this inhibitory activity has been however attributed to EPA, although DHA is generally ingested in similar amounts and some studies have shown the efficacy of pure DHA intake. We report *in vitro* studies comparing platelet enrichment with EPA or DHA, revealing that DHA is rather more potent than EPA in inhiting platelet aggregation. Their mechanism of action differs entirely, especially at the phospholipid level. Whereas EPA is released from phospholipid subclasses similarly to endogenous arachidonic acid, and competes for the formation of thromboxane A$_2$, DHA not released virtually but efficiently transfered from phosphatidylcholine to phosphatidylenolamine during platelet activation. Concomitantly to this peculiar phospholipid metabolism, DHA also decreases thromboxane formation from endogenous arachidonic acid and thromboxane-induced aggregation as well as its specific binding to platelet membranes.
We conclude that an original metabolism of DHA at the membrane phospholipid level could explain most of its biological activity in platelets.

Introduction

Since the epidemiological studies by Dyeberg *et al.* [1] showing a very low frequency of cardiovascular diseases in Eskimos, number of investigations have confirmed the potential protective effect of fish fat against atherosclerosis and thrombosis [2]. This may be due to beneficial effects on plasma lipoproteins [3] as well as on blood and vascular cells involved in these pathological processes [4].

Among these cells, platelets and endothelial cells have been well investigated. One feature concerns the inhibition of thromboxane A_2 formation form platelet arachidonic acid (AA) by EPA [5] while the latter is converted into thromboxane A_3 devoid of pro-aggregatory and vasoconstrictor properties [6]. In contrast, the vascular endothelium converts EPA into prostaglandin I_3 which shares the biological activity of prostaglandin I_2 (prostacyclin) [7]. It is then assumed that overall, the balance between thromboxane and prostacyclin is shifted towards its anti-aggregatory and vasodilating potential, which could explain the beneficial effect of fish fat intakes in preventing atherosclerosis and thrombosis.

EPA is also believed to reduce the activity of blood cells involved in inflammation which might contribute in these pathological processes. This refers in particular to leukocytes and their production of leukotriene B_4, a potent chemotactic agent, and of platelet-activating factor (PAF), a pro-inflammatory phospholipid acting at several stages of the inflammatory process. Leukotriene B_4 production is decreased and partially replaced by leukotriene B5 which is much less active than its analogue B_4 [8],while PAF generation is markedly reduced [9].

Although DHA is consumed in similar amount as EPA in various fish fat preparations, few investigations have been performed to precise its contribution in the effects observed [10]. These investigations concern mainly platelets and reveal that DHA could be even more potent than EPA in preventing platelet aggregation [11, 12].

We report here that the mechanism of action for platelet inhibition by DHA differs entirely from that of EPA, with special reference to platelet phospholipid metabolism.

Phospholipid metabolism

When studied *in vitro* via the Lands pathway (acylation/deacylation) [13], EPA and DHA, pre-coated onto albumin, are efficiently taken up by human platelets. The main unesterified polyunsaturated fatty acid of the normal human plasma, linoleic acid (LA) and AA, are able to compete with the uptake of EPA and DHA. The study was done in the presence of ten fold higher concentration of LA and equal concentration of AA to simulate the physiological ratio between these latter fatty acids in plasma. Although both LA and AA reduced the total incorporation of EPA and DHA into platelet lipid pools. AA proved to be more active than LA, suggesting that the closest configuration off AA, compared to EPA and DHA, is crucial for competing at the uptake stage. Under the above mentioned conditions, 90 % of EPA and 80 % of DHA are acylated in glycerophospholipids, the remaining being acylated in neutral lipids, mainly triacyglycerols, especially for DHA [14]. Looking at the glycerophospholipid class distribution of each of both EPA and DHA, we found a substantial difference in which EPA was mainly acylated into phosphatidylcholine (PC) (> 60 %) with only 10 % in phosphalidylethanolamine (PE) whereas DHA was distributed according to 40 and 30 %, respectively. This agrees with the general assumption that DHA is preferentially located in PE of most tissues [15].

In the presence of aggregating agents inducing platelet phospholipase activities like thrombin and the calcium ionophore A23187, EPA is released from total phospholipids but DHA is not. The percentage release of EPA is quite similar to that of AA from its endogenous pool. At the level of each glycerophospholipid, a very marked difference could be observed between both Ω-3 fatty acid. EPA behaves quite similarly as endogenous AA with a release from PC and secondarily from phosphatidylinositol (PI). The release from PI might be not relevant since the incorporation of EPA into PI appears to be very low *in vivo* [16]. Unexpectingly, DHA is released markedly from PC and reacylated reciprocally into PE [17]. The reciprocal reacylation of DHA into PE is likely to explain the absence of release observed when examined at the total glycerophospholipid level.

Oxygenated metabolism

Subsequently to its release from membrane phospholipids, EPA is efficiently oxygenated via the 12-lipoxygenase pathway, and to a lesser entent via the cyclooxygenase/thromboxane synthase pathway [18]. The efficient oxygenation can occur because of the simultaneous released AA which is concomitantly converted into its lipoxygenase product, 12-hydroperoxyeicosatetraenoic acid [12-HPETE]. This peroxyde potentiates very markedly the oxygenation of EPA [19, 20]. In addition to the reduced thromboxane

A_2 formation, the production of substantial amount of the end-lipoxygenase product of EPA (12-HEPE) could contribute to platelet inhibition in antagonizing thromboxane A_2 – induced platelet aggregation [21, 22].

In contrast, DHA virtually is not oxygenated, although its convertion by platelet lipoxygenase is also potentiated efficiently by AA, presumably via 12-HPETE [23]. This is likely due to the absence of its release from membrane phospholipids and suggests, that the marked transfer observed from PC to PE under platelet stimulation occurs without substantial liberation.

Simultaneously the oxygenation of endogenous AA into prostanoids is decreased in EPA- or DHA-rich platelets while the lipoxygenation of AA is not altered [23]. The cyclooxygenase and thromboxane synthase being membrane bound enzymes whereas the lipoxygenase is cytosolic, this may indicate that EPA and DHA might inhibit the enzyme at the level of membrane lipid-protein interactions.

Conclusion

From these results we may conclude that the two main polyunsaturated fatty acids from fish fat are both efficient inhibitors of platelet function *in vitro,* but act through entirely different mechanism. Whereas EPA competes with the endogenous AA at several stages, DHA prevents platelet aggregation by different ways, among these the specific transfer between PC and PE could be important to account for.

References

1. Dyeberg J, Bang HO, Stoffersen E *et al*. Eicosapentaenoic acid and prevention of thrombosis and atherosclerosis. Lancet 1978; ii : 117-19.
2. Leaf A and Weber PC. Cardiovascular effects of n-3 fatty acids. New Engl J Med 1988; 318 : 549-57.
3. Goodnight SH, Harris SH, Connor WE *et al*. Polyunsaturated fatty acids, hyperlipidemia and thrombosis. Artheriosclerosis 1982; 2 : 87-113.
4. Ross R. The pathogenesis of atherosclerosis – an update. New Engl J Med 1986; 314 : 488-500.
5. Siess W, Roth P, Scherer B *et al*. Platelet membrane fatty acids, platelet aggregation, and thromboxane formation during a mackerel diet. Lancet 1980; i : 441-4.

6. Needleman Ph, Raz A, Minkes Ms *et al.* Triene prostaglandins : prostacyclin and thromboxane biosynthesis. A unique biological properties. Proc Natl Sci USA 1979; 76 : 744-8.

7. Fisher S, Weber PC, Prostaglandin I₃ is formed *in vivo* in man after dietary eicosapentaenoic acid. Nature 1984; 307 : 165-8.

8. Terano T, Salmon JA, Moncada S. Biosynthesis and biological activity of leukotriene B₅. Protaglandins 1984; 27 : 217-32.

9. Pickett WE, Nytko D, Dondero-Zahn C *et al.* The effect of endogenous eicosapentaenoic acid on PMN leukotriène and PAF biosynthesis. Prostagland Leuk Med 1986; 23 : 135-40.

10. Lagarde M. Metabolism of fatty acids by platelets and the function of various metabolites in mediating platelet function. Progr Lipid Res 1988; 27 : 135-52.

11. V Schacky C, Weber PC. Metabolism and effect on platelet function of the purified eicosapentaenoic and docosahexaenoid acids in humans. J Clin Invest 1985; 76 : 2446-50.

12. Croset M, Lagarde M. *In vitro* incorporation and metabolism of eicosapentaenoic and docosahexaenoic acids in human platelets. Effect on aggregation. Throm Haemost 1986; 56 : 57-62.

13. Lands Wem, Heart P. Control of fatty acid composition in glycerol phospholipids J Am Oil Chem Soc 1965; 43 : 290-5.

14. Hajarine M, Lagarde M. Studies on polyenoic acid incorporation into human platelet lipid stores : interactions with linoleic and arachidonic acids. Biochim Biophys Acta 1986; 877 : 299-304.

15. Tinoco. Dietary requirements and functions of α-linolenic acid in animals. Progr Lipid Res 1982; 21 : 1-45.

16. Galloway JH, Cortwright IJ, Woodcock BE *et al.* Effects of dietary fish oil supplementation on the fatty acid composition of human platelet membrane : demonstration of selectivity in the incorporation of eicosapentaenoic acid into membrane phospholipids. Clin Sci 1985; 68 : 449-54.

17. Hajarine M, Lagarde M. Liberation and oxygenation of polyenoic acids in stimulated platelets. Biochimic 1988; 70 : 1749-58.

18. Lagarde M, Drouot B, Guichardant M *et al.* *In vitro* incorporation and metabolism of some eicosaenoic acids in platelets. Effect on arachidonic acid oxygenation. Biochim Biophys Acta 1985; 833 : 52-8.

19. Morita I, Takahashi R, Saito Y *et al.* Stimulation of eicosapentaenoic acid metabolism in washed human platelets by 12-hydroperoxy-eicosatetraenoic acid. J Biol Chem 1983; 258 : 10297-99.

20. Croset M, Lagarde M. Enhancement of eicosaenoic acid lipoxygenation in human platelets by 12-hydroperoxy derivative of arachidonic acid. Lipids 1985; 20 : 743-50.

21. Croset M, Lagarde M. Stereospecific inhibition of PGH₂-induced platelet aggregation by lipoxygenase products of icosaenoic acids. Biochem Biophys Res Commun 1983; 112 ; 879-83.

22. Coene MC, Bult H, Claeys M *et al.* Inhibition of rabbit platelet activation by lipoxygenase products of arachidonic and linoleic acids. Thromb Res 1986; 42 : 205-14.

23. Croset M, Guichardant M, Lagard M. Different metabolic behavior of long chain Ω-3 polyunsaturated fatty acids in human platelets. Biochim Biophys Acta 1988; 961 : 262-9.

Fish oil and blood-vessel wall interactions. Eds P.M. Vanhoutte, Ph. Douste-Blazy.
John Libbey Eurotext, Paris © 1991, pp. 69-79.

7

Fish oils and growth factors for vascular smooth muscle cells

P.L. Fox, P.E. DiCorleto

*Department of Vascular Cell Biology and Atherosclerosis,
Cleveland Clinic Research Institute, 9500 Euclid Avenue,
Cleveland, Ohio 44195, USA.*

Abstract

Epidemiological evidence suggests that ingestion of a diet rich in fish and fish oils may be related to reduced incidence of atherosclerosis and other cardiovascular diseases. Studies using several animal models of experimental atherosclerosis, including dogs, rats, pigs, and non-human primates, have shown that fish oils significantly reduce intimal hyperplasia in a number of arterial vessels. The results of similar experiments using rabbit models are inconclusive. The effect of fish oils on restenosis after percutaneous coronary angioplasty has also been investigated. In two recent studies, fish oils have significantly reduced restenosis, however, in two other studies this reduction is not observed.
The mechanisms by which fish oils elicit their proposed beneficial effects have not been elucidated, but two areas that have been actively investigated are lipoprotein metabolism and platelet reactivity. We have suggested an alternate mechanism, that fish oils reduce intimal hyperplasia by inhibiting the production of growth factors for smooth muscle cells. On such growth factor, platelet-derived, growth factor has been shown to stimulate both migration and proliferation of cultured smooth muscle cells. Platelet-derived growth factor is also the principle smooth muscle cells mitogen in human serum and is secreted by several vascular cells. In particular, endothelial cells from all species cultured to date constitutively secrete platelet-derived growth factor at a high rate. Secretion of platelet-derived growth factor into the intima may thus play a role in the smooth muscle cells proliferation that is hallmark of the atherosclerotic lesion. We have shown that emulsions of Ω-3 fatty acid* containing 30 % Ω-3 fatty acid inhibit the production of platelet-derived growth factor by confluent cultures of bovine aortic endothelial cells.

(*) Maxepa [®].

Safflower oil, containing primarily Ω-6 polyunsaturated fatty acids, has less than one-tenth of the inhibitory activity of Ω-3 fatty acid and peanut oil, containing mostly saturated and monounsaturated lipids is inactive. The inhibitory activity of Ω-3 fatty acid is inhibited by the antioxidants vitamin E and butylated hydroxytoluene, suggesting that the inhibitor lipid may be an oxidized molecule or that cellular oxidative processes may be critical for the activity. We have speculated that differences in levels of lipid oxidation may be in part responsible for the discrepancies observed in animal studies and clinical trials.

The observation that diets enriched in fish and fish oils are correlated with a reduced incidence of cardiovascular disease in man, has stimulated two decades of investigations aimed at elucidating the underlying mechanisms. These studies, whether in cell culture, in experimental animal models, or in clinical trials, have focused primarily on two aspects of vascular biology : 1) lipoprotein metabolism, specifically the cholesterol – and triglyceride – lowering effects of fish oils, and 2) coagulation, specifically the effects of Ω-3 fatty acids on eicosanoid metabolism and platelet aggregation. Recently, we have suggested an alternative mechanism through which fish oils could mediate their beneficial effects, i.e., by inhibiting the release of specific growth factors that stimulate the growth of vascular smooth muscle cells. This cell is the primary proliferative cell involved in intimal thickening, a hallmark of the occlusive atherosclerotic lesion. In this report, the results from laboratories and others that have led to the formulation of this hypothesis will be described.

Reduction of Intimal Hyperplasia by Fish Oils

Direct measurements of the effects of dietary fish oils on intimal thickening have been reported by laboratories working with several animal models of atherosclerosis. The first report that fish oils reduced intimal hyperplasia was that by Landymore *et al.* [1] who observed that cod liver oil markedly reduced intimal thickening in autogenous vein grafts implanted as arterial bypasses in cholesterol-fed dogs. Interestingly, they found that fish oils did not alter any platelet parameters, including platelet counts and prothrombin time, suggesting that the observed vessel response to the diet did not depend on interactions with platelets. Cahill *et al.* [2] confirmed this result using a similar animal model; they showed that Ω-3 fatty acid*, like cod liver oil, also prevented intimal thickening in vein grafts implanted in dogs. Like

---

(*) Maxepa ®

Landymore's group, they also found that the fish oil did not affect coagulation parameters, nor did it alter vessel prostacyclin production, serum lipid levels, or the number of hepatic low density lipoprotein receptors. They did, however, report a small but significant reduction in serum thromboxane levels. Sarris *et al* [3], using a similar canine vein graft model, recently showed that Ω-3 fatty acid, with or without aspirin, was significantly more effective than aspirin alone at reducing intimal thickening. In a related animal model, Casali *et al.* [4] demonstrated that a diet of fish and fish oils improved the patency of synthetic vascular grafts in dogs. They did not, however, directly measure intimal thickening in these grafts. The effect of fish oils on atherosclerosis in a rat model of cardiac transplantation was studied by Sarris *et al.* [5]. Lewis rats that received (in the presence of cyclosporine) heterotopic hearts from Brown-Norway donors were found to develop severe coronary atherosclerosis that was mitigated by Super Ω-3 fatty acid* but not by safflower oil, a polyunsaturated lipid that is rich in Ω-6 fatty acids. The effects of fish oils on intimal thickening of native vessels, rather than implanted grafts, have also been investigated. Luminal encroachment in coronary arteries of cholesterol-fed pigs was substantially inhibited by the addition of cod liver oil to the diet [6]. This result was confirmed for multiple coronary arteries as well as several regions of the aorta [7]. Studies on the effects of fish oils on the development of atherosclerosis and intimal hyperplasia in rabbit models have led to conflicting results. Fish oil was shown to reduce significantly the area of the involved plaque region in cholesterol-fed rabbits, however, the effects on intimal thickening were not determined [8]. Hearn *et al.* [9] reported mixed results with respect to the effect of Ω-3 fatty acid on intimal hyperplasia in rabbits who underwent balloon de-endothelialization of the aorta and iliac arteries while consuming a cholesterol- and peanut oil-enriched diet. They reported a mild sparing of the lumen diameter in the iliacs, but thickening of the aorta wall (although without reduction of the overall luminal area). Thiery and Seidel [10] reported that Ω-3 fatty acid enhances lesion area in cholesterol-fed rabbits (but lumen diameters were not measured). Finally, two groups have reported that fish oils Ω-3 fatty acid or menhaden oil) do not alter the surface extent of atherosclerosis or lesion thickness in Watanabe heritable hyperlipidemic rabbits [11, 12]. Using the hypercholesterolemic rat model of atherosclerosis, Rogers and Karnovsky [13] have shown that Ω-3 fatty acid enhances monocyte adhesion to the vessel wall, and augments fatty streak formation. The effect of fish oil on atherosclerosis in non-human primates has been reported in a single study. Davis *et al.* [14] showed that menhaden oil reduced lesion area in the aorta and carotid artery of cholesterol-fed rhesus monkeys. The control

---

(*) Super Maxepa ®.

treatment consisted of equivalent amounts of coconut oil, which is known to accelerate atherogenesis, and thus it is not clear if the observed results resulted from a specific beneficial property of the fish oil, or simply from a decrease in the saturated fatty acid content in the diet.

The apparent discrepancies in several of the animal studies have not yet been resolved, but there are clearly many variables that must be considered. Some of these critical variables are : the specific animal model of atheros-clerosis (and especially the physical disruption and/or diet used to induce lesions), the dose and type of fish oil used (the quantity of Ω-3 fatty acids, anti-oxidants, and minor unidentified components, may all contribute to the activity), the duration of the fish oil treatment, the methods employed for quantitation of atherosclerotic lesions, and the nature of the control treatment to which the fish oil treatment is compared. It may be significant that in both studies in which atherosclerosis was reported to be enhanced by fish oils, parameters other than intimal thickening were measured [10, 13].

The effect of fish oils on restenosis of coronary arteries after percutaneous transluminal angioplasty was examined in several recent clinical trials. This procedure has a very high initial success rate, but the long-term benefit is compromised by recurring restenosis in approximately one-third of the ves-sels, the failure generally occuring within six months. Dehmer et al. [15] reported that Ω-3 fatty acid reduced the early restenosis rate from 36 % of the lesions in the control group to 16 % in the treatment group A nearly identical reduction in lesion restenosis, from 35 % in controls to 19 % in the treatment group, was reported by Milner et al. [16] in patients receiving Promega [®]. These intriguing results, however, were not confirmed by two other recent reports. Grigg et al. [17] reported similar rates of restenosis between a treatment group that received Ω-3 fatty acid (31 % of lesions). Likewise, Reis et al. [18] did not observe significant differences in restenosis in a treatment group given either Promega [®] or ethyl esters of fatty acids extracted from fish oils (32 % of lesions), and the control group receiving 12 g/day of olive oil (23 % of lesions).

The discrepancies in these clinical studies are not likely due to the ancillary therapies since all treatment and control groups received anti-platelet agents and calcium channel blockers (although according to differing regimens). The dose and source of the fish oil also does not readily explain the dis-crepant results; in terms of the actual amount of Ω-3 fatty acids administered, the effective treatments contained 5.4 and 4.5 g/day, while the ineffective treatments contained 3.0 and 6.0 g/day. However, one of the two treatment groups in the Reis study received fatty acids ethyl esters whose activity has not been established in the animal models, and the results from each group were not independently reported.

Growth Factors and Atherosclerosis

Balloon catheter injury of arteries, in several animal models, results in rapid accumulation of smooth muscle cells to form an occlusive lesion that resembles an atherosclerotic plaque. Ross and Glomset [19], to explain this observation, have suggested the "response to injury hypothesis of atherosclerosis" in which removal of the endothelium by physical, chemical, or immunological injury causes platelet adherence to the subendothelial surface, subsequent release from the platelets of growth factors for vascular smooth muscle cells, and finally migration of smooth muscle cells into the intima and subsequent proliferation. Growth factors (or mitogens) are hormone-like proteins that bind to specific receptors on target cells, initiating a cascade of events that culminates in mitosis and cell replication. Ross and coworkers have isolated and identified the principal human serum mitogen for vascular smooth muscle cells, platelet-derived growth factor. Platelet-derived growth factor binds to specific, high affinity surface receptors on smooth muscle cells (as well as on fibroblasts and other mesenchymal cells), and in addition to causing cell proliferation platelet-derived growth factor is also a smooth muscle cells chemoattractant. A scenario thus can be imagined in which an elevated concentration of platelet-derived growth factor in the intima stimulates inward migration and proliferation of media smooth muscle cells.

During the last decade attention has been focused on both the function as well as the potential sources of platelet-derived growth factor in the arterial environment. DiCorleto and Bowen-Pope [20] have shown that endothelial cells *in vitro* secrete platelet-derived growth factor in amounts sufficient to stimulate the proliferation of cultured smooth muscle cells. Endothelial cells cultured from all major vessels, and from all species examined to date, secrete PDGF into their medium. The process in constitutive, i.e. exogenous stimulation of the cells is not required; however, factors related to arterial injury stimulate the release of the growth factor. For example, certain members of the coagulation cascade, including thrombin and Factor Xa, increase the rate of synthesis of platelet-derived growth factor by cultured endothelial cells up to 10-fold [21]. In addition, several agents that mortally injure cultured bovine aortic endothelial cells, including bacterial lipopylysaccharide, cause the release of a large burst of platelet-derived growth factor, presumably from dying cells [22]. These observations have to a modified version of the "response to injury" hypothesis, in which injury to the endothelium leads to release of growth factors from vessel wall cells rather than from circulating platelets *(Figure 1)*. According to this model, the presence, not

73

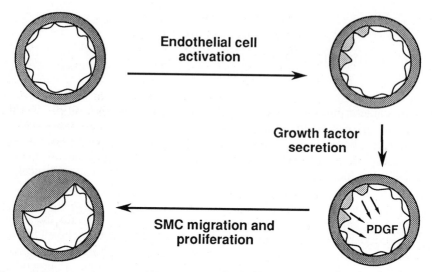

Figure 1. The Modified Response to Injury Hypothesis of Atherosclerosis. Schematic showing the proposed relationship of endothelial cell activation to lesion formation. Abbreviations : platelet-derived growth factor (PDGF), smooth muscle cell (SMC).

absence, of the endothelium is necessary for the expression of its pro-atherogenic properties.

Evidence that endothelial cells are involved in Smooth muscle cells proliferation *in vivo* is largely circumstantial. Until the late stages of atherosclerosis, endothelial denudation is not observed, thus suggesting that platelet aggregation may not be required. Furthermore, Reidy and Silver [23] have shown that a shallow, defined injury to the aorta that does not cause medial injury, results in platelet aggregation but no intimal thickening. This result indicates that platelet products alone are not sufficient to cause smooth muscle cells proliferation. Finally, intimal hyperplasia in many circumstances correlates with regions of endothelialization, for example at the anastomoses of synthetic vascular grafts.

Direct *in vivo* measurements of growth factor production by endothelial cells or other vascular cells are not easily accomplished due to the technical problems. However, measurements of the transcriptional activity of the genes encoding growth factors can be measured in freshly isolated tissue by extracting the mRNA and determining the level of the specific transcripts by Northern analysis. The expression of platelet-derived growth factor B-chain mRNA (one of the two polypeptides forming human platelet-derived growth factor) is at least 10-fold lower in endothelium freshly scraped from human umbilical vein or bovine aorta than in the comparable cultured endothelial cells. Furthermore, B-chain mRNA is present in 5-fold greater amounts in human carotid artery lesions than in normal artery, although the cell responsible for the production of platelet-derived growth factor has not been specifically identified. These results raise the interesting possibility that endothelial cells may be "activated", either in response to pathological stimuli *in vivo,* or simply by the transition from the physiological state *in vivo* to the more rigorous *in vitro* condition. If this is the case, then studies on the conditions that inactivate cultured endothelical cells i.e. lead to the reduction of growth factor production, may give insights into the physiological conditions required to maintain the endothelium in the "inactive" or anti-atherogenic state.

Vascular cells other than endothelial cells may also synthesize and secrete growth factors into the arterial wall. Several laboratories have shown that human peripheral blood monocytes, activated *in vitro* by bacterial lipopolysaccharide or by immune complexes, secrete PDGF. In addition, smooth muscle cells themselves, under certain circumstances produce growth factors. Smooth muscle cells cultured from the aorta of rat pups secrete significantly more platelet-derived growth factor than smooth muscle cells isolated from adult rats, suggesting that a normal function of platelet-derived growth factor may be related to blood vessel development. Cultured smooth muscle cells derived from intimal lesions of mechanically injured rat arteries also produce more platelet-derived growth factor than medial smooth muscle cells from uninjured arteries. This results is supported by a study reported by Wilcox *et al.* [26] in which *in situ* hybridization histochemistry is used to determine the *in vivo* location and identity of atherosclerotic lesion cells expressing the genes for the A-chain and B-chain of platelet-derived growth factor. Endothelial cells and intimal smooth muscle cells express both gene transcripts, but medial smooth muscle cells and macrophages show little of either. These results suggest that smooth muscle cells derived growth factors may stimulate their own growth in an autocrine fashion, similar to the mechanism postulated for the uncontrolled cell proliferation characteristic of certain tumors.

Fish Oils and Growth Factors for Smooth Muscle Cells

We have investigated the effects of plasma lipoproteins on growth factor production by endothelial cells. Certain modified lipoproteins, including low density lipoprotein (LDL) that is modified by acetylation, and LDL that is oxidized by *in vitro* free radical oxidation, inhibit PDGF production by up to 75 % compared to lipoprotein-free controls [27]. The inhibitory activity

75

of both lipoproteins is directly related to the level of lipid peroxidation as measured as thiobarbituric acid-reactive substances. The solvent-extracted lipids from oxidized LDL also inhibit growth factor production. Since these results, and those from several other laboratories, clearly show that oxidized lipids dramatically influence endothelial cells function, we have begun to investigate the interactions with endothelial cells of another easily oxidizable lipid mixture, the marine lipids rich in Ω-3 fatty acids. In these experiments a stable emulsion of containing approximately 30 % Ω-3 fatty acids, is prepared by sonication with egg for dimyristoyl phosphatidylcholine [28]. Ω-3 fatty acid emulsions inhibit the production of platelet-derived growth factor by at least 70 % in confluent cultures of bovine aortic endothelial cells *(Figure 2)*. Cod liver oil, containing approximately 20 % Ω-3 fatty acids, is nearly as inhibitory. Safflower oil, a polyunsaturated lipid containing only trace amounts of Ω-3 fatty acids, also inhibits growth factor production but with a potency 10 to 20 times less than the fish oils. Peanut oil, containing

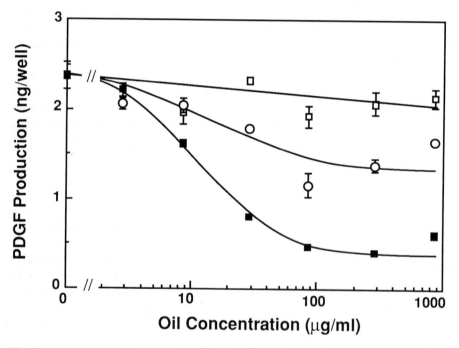

Figure 2. The Inhibition of Endothelial Cell Production of Platelet-Derived Growth Factor by Fish Oil. Emulsions of Ω-3 fatty acid (■), safflower oil (o), and peanut oil (□) were prepared by sonication with egg phosphatidylcholine. The emulsions were incubated for 72 h with confluent cultures of bovine aortic EC, and platelet-derived growth factor (PDGF) in the conditioned medium was assayed by a specific radioreceptor assay.

primarily saturated and monounsaturated fatty acids, completely lacks inhibitory activity. The inhibitory activity of the fish oils is for the most part specific since the rate of overal protein synthesis, as measured by incorporation of radiolabeled leucine into protein, is unaltered. This same result also indicates that the inhibition of growth factor production is not due to a toxic effect of the lipid on the endothelial cells cultures.

The identify of the lipid(s) in fish oils that specifically inhibits platelet-derived growth factor production has not been determined. A candidate molecule is cholesterol which is a minor component of most fish oil extracts, comprising up to 0.5 % of the total mass. Incubation of endothelial cells with cholesterol/albumine complexes results in sufficient lipid-loading to increase the cellular cholesterol content by 50 %, however, the inhibitory activity of cholesterol is only marginal and cannot account for the activity of fish oils [27]. The inhibitory activity of Ω-3 fatty acid is inhibited by the addition of anti-oxidants to the cultures; vitamin E is partially inhibitory while butylated hydroxytoluene is nearly completely suppressive [28]. It is thus clear that oxidative processes play a critical role in this particular activity of fish oils, but it has not yet been determined if the inhibitor molecule is itself an oxidized lipid, or if oxidative processes within the cell are required for the expression of the inhibitory activity. If the inhibitor is a minor component of fish oil, e.g., and oxidized lipid, then identification of this lipid should result in more potent, and perhaps more tolerable, treatments. Furthermore, it is certainly possible that differences in the level of oxidation of fish oil and the presence of anti-oxidants in the extract, may contribute to the discrepancies observed in both the animal studies and the clinical trials.

The effects of fish oils on the release of growth factor activity from other cells has been recently reported. Eicosapentaenoic acid and docosahexaenoic acid, Ω-3 fatty acid that are major constituents of fish oils, inhibit the relase of unidentified mitogens from ADP-stimulated platelets and from monocyte-derived macrophages *in vitro* [29]. In addition, Sarris *et al.* [3] have reported that implantation of autologous vein grafts in hypercholesterolemic dogs caused increased serum mitogenic activity that was mitigated by dietary fish oils. Although the cellular source of the mitogen is not established with certainty, the authors speculate that the fish oil-mediated inhibition of mitogen release from platelets, and not changes in lipoprotein or eicosanoid metabolism, is responsible for the anti-atherogenic properties of fish oils.

Investigation of the effects of fish oils on the metabolism of vascular cells remains in its infancy. The functional changes induced by fish oils must be better understood at the cellular level, and the ensuing responses, especially the secretion of paracrine agents that alter nearby cells, must be identified. Finally, the identity of the lipid(s) responsible for the cellular responses, and the mechanisms underlying these responses, also must be determined. These investigations at the cellular level should provide important insights into, and suggest new directions for, *in vivo* studies on the role of fish oils in cardiovascular disease.

References

1. Landymore RW, Kinley CE, Cooper JH *et al.,* Cod-liver oil in the prevention of intimal hyperplasia in autogenous vein grafts for arterial bypass. J Thorac Cardiovasc Surg 1985; 89 : 351-7.

2. Cahill PD, Sarris GE, Cooper AD *et al.* Inhibition of vein graft intimal thickening by eicosapentaenoic acid : Reduced thromboxane production without change in lipoprotein levels or low-density lipoproptein receptor density. J Vasc Surg 1988; 7 : 108-18.

3. Sarris GE, Fann JI, Sokoloff MH *et al.* Mechanisms responsible for inhibition of vein-graft arteriosclerosis by fish oil. Circulation 1988; 80 : I-109-23.

4. Casali RE, Hale JA, LeNarz L *et al.* Improved graft patency associated with altered platelet function induced by marine fatty acids in dogs. J Surg Res 1986; 40 : 6-12.

5. Sarris GE, Mitchell RS, Billingham ME *et al.* Inhibition of accelerated cardiac allograft arteriocleroclerosis by fish oil. J Thorac Cardiovasc Surg 1989; 97 : 841-55.

6. Weiner BH, Ockene IS, Levine PH *et al.* Inhibition of Atherosclerosis by cod-liver oil in a hyperlipidemic swine model. N Eng J Med 1986; 315 : 841-6.

7. Kim DN, Ho H-T, Lawrence DA *et al.* Modification of lipoprotein patterns and retardation of atherogenesis by a fish oil supplement to a hyperlipidemic diet for swine. Atherosclerosis 1989; 76 : 35-54.

8. Zhu B-Q, Smith DL, Sievers RE *et al.* Inhibition of atherosclerosis by fish oil in cholesterol-fed rabbits. J Am Coll Cardiol 1988; 12 : 1073-78.

9. Hearn JA, Shoutas DS, Robinson KA *et al.* Marine lipid concentrate and atherosclerosis in the rabbit model. Atherosclerosis 1989; 75 : 39-47.

10. Thiery J, Seidel D. Fish oil feeding results in an enhancement of cholesterol-induced atherosclerosis in rabbits. Atherosclerosis 1987; 63 : 53-6.

11. Clubb FJ, Schmitz JM, butler MM *et al.* Effect of dietary omega-3 fatty acid on serum lipids, platelet function, and atherosclerosis in Watanabe heritable hyperlipidemic rabbits. Atherosclerosis 1989; 9 : 529-37.

12. Rich S, Miller JF, Charous S *et al.* Development of atherosclerosis in genetically hyperlipidemic rabbits during chronic fish-oil ingestion. Atherosclerosis 1989; 9 : 189-94.

13. Rogers KA, Karnovsky MJ. Dietary fish oil enhances monocyte adhesion and fatty streak formation in the hypercholesterolemic rat. Am J Pathol 1988; 132 : 382-8.

14. Davis HR, Bridenstine RT, Vesselinovitch D *et al.* Fish oil inhibits development of atherosclerosis in rhesus monkeys. Atherosclerosis 1987; 7 : 441-9.

15. Dehmer GJ, Popma JJ, Van den Berg EK *et al.* Reduction in the rate of early restenosis after coronary angioplasty by a diet supplemented with n-3 fatty acids. N Eng J Med 1988; 319 : 733-40.

16. Milner MR, Gaffino RA, Leffingwell A *et al*. Usefulness of fish oil supplements in preventing clinical evidence of restenosis after percutaneous transluminal coronary angioplasty. Am J Cardiol 1989; 64 : 294-9.

17. Grigg LE, Kay TWH, Valentine PA *et al*. Determinants of restenosis an lack of effect of dietary supplementation with eicosapentaenoic acid on the incidence of coronary artery restenosis after angioplasty. J Am Coll Cardiol 1989; 13 : 665-72.

18. Reis GJ, Boucher TM, Sipperly ME *et al*. Randomised trial of fish oil for prevention of restenosis after coronary angioplasty. Lancet 1989; ii : 177-81.

19. Ross R, Glomset JA. Atherosclerosis and the arterial smooth muscle cell. Science 1973; 180 : 1332-9.

20. DiCorleto PE, Bowen-Pope DF. Cultured endothelial cells produce a platelet-derived growth factor-like protein. Proc Natl Acad Sci USA 1983; 80 : 1919-23.

21. Harlan JM, Thompson PJ, Ross RR *et al*. α-Trombin induces release of platelet-derived growth factor-like molecule(s) by cultured endothelial cells. H Cell Biol 1986; 103 : 1129-33.

22. Fox PL, DiCorleto PE. Regulation of production of a platelet-derived growth factor-like protein by cultured bovine aortic endothelial cells. J Cell Physiol 1984; 121 : 298-308.

23. Reidy MA, Silver M. Endothelial regeneration. VII.Lack of intimal proliferation after defined injury to rat aorta. 1985; 118 : 173-7.

24. Barrett TB, Gajdusek CM, Schwartz SM *et al*. Expression of the *sis* gene by endothelial cells in culture and *in vivo*. Proc Natl Acad Sci USA 1984; 81 : 6772-4.

25. Barrett TB, Benditt EP. *Sis* (platelet-derived growth factor B chain) gene transcript levels are elevated in human atherosclerotic lesions compared to normal artery. Proc Natl Acad Sci USA 1987; 84 : 1099-1103.

26. Wilcox JN, Smith KM, Williams LT *et al*. Platelet-derived growth factor mRNA detection in human atherosclerotic plaques by in situ hydridization. J Clin Invest 1988; 82 : 1134-43.

27. Fox PL, Chisolm GM, DiCorleto PE. Lipoprotein-mediated inhibition of endothelial cell production of platelet-derived growth factor-like protein depends on free radical lipid peroxidation. J Biol Chem 1987; 262 : 6046-54.

28. Fox PL, DiCorleto PE. Fish oils inhibit endothelial cell production of platelet-derived growth factor-like protein. Science 1988; 241 : 453-6.

29. Smith DL, Willis AL, Nguyen N *et al*. Eskimo plasma constituents, dihomo-γ-linolenic acid, eicosapentaenoic acid and docosahexaenoic acid inhibit the release of atherogenic mitogens. Lipids 1989; 24 : 70-5.

Fish oil and blood-vessel wall interactions. Eds P.M. Vanhoutte, Ph. Douste-Blazy.
John Libbey Eurotext, Paris © 1991, pp. 81-88.

8

Effects of dietary fish oil in experimental models of atherosclerosis

B. Greenberg

*Division of Cardiology, L-462, Oregon Health Sciences University,
3181 SW Sam Jackson Park Road, Portland,
OR 97201-3098. (503) 279-8750, USA.*

Abstract

Experimental animal models of atherosclerosis have proven to be of great value in assessing the anti-atherogenic properties of dietary fish oil. These models enable investigators to detect beneficial actions in a much shorter period of time than would be possible in humans. In addition, the confounding influences that are invariably present in human studies can be avoided. There is evidence that dietary fish oil can inhibit the development of atherosclerosis in vein graft in dogs, in the aorta of some rabbit models, in swine coronary arteries and in a variety of arteries in non human primates. The mechanism(s) responsible for these protective effects us uncertain, but alterations in plasma lipids and lipoprotein do not appear to be sufficient to account for all of the changes that have been seen. The findings from studies done in experimental animal models are likely to be highly relevant to humans in whom atherosclerosis remains a leading cause of death.

The possibility that Ω-3 fatty acids might have anti-atherogenic properties was first suggested by epidemiologic surveys which reported a low prevalence of coronary artery disease in populations that consumed a diet rich in fish or sea mammals [1, 2]. In support of these observations, there is a rapidly expanding body of information from studies of both cell biology and human metabolism which indicates that dietary fish oil can favorably influence many of the pathways that are believed to be important in the development of atherosclerosis and its clinical sequelae of ischemia and in-

Table I. Biologic effects of fish oil

1. Plasma lipid and lipoprotein concentrations [3]
2. Platelet function and platelet-vessel wall interactions [4, 5, 6]
3. Eicosanoid formation [5, 6]
4. Leukocyte function [7]
5. Cytokine and growth factor production [8]
6. Endothelium-derived relaxation factor (EDRF activity) [9]
7. Arterial pressure [10]
8. Blood viscosity [11]

farction [3, 11]. Some of the relevant biologic effects of fish oil are listed in *Table I.*

The results of these studies, though provocative and intriguing, do not provide direct evidence that there is a cause and effect relationship between dietary fish oil and protection from atherosclerotic disease. A major step towards reaching that conclusion comes from studies performed in animal models of experimental atherosclerosis. Such studies are extremely valuable in that they can provide information regarding efficacy in a relatively short period of time compared to trials in humans. Confounding influences such as co-existent disease, other drug therapy, and environmental factors that complicate studies in patients can be avoided. Experimental animal models also provide unique opportunities to investigate possible mechanisms responsible for the beneficial effects as well as to recognize potential toxic effects of therapy. The purpose of this review is to describe and summarize the results of published studies evaluating the effects of dietary fish oil in experimental animals models of atherosclerosis.

Effects of fish oil on intimal hyperplasia in vein grafts

One of the earliest studies using an experimental animal model to evaluate the effects of dietary fish oil on a form of atherosclerotic disease was published by Landymore *et al.* in 1986 [12]. In this study, 3 groups of dogs were fed a highly atherogenic 2 % cholesterol diet and the development of intimal hyperplasia was assessed in segments of external jugular vein which had been juxtaposed in the femoral artery. One group received diet alone, another group received dipyridamole (2.5 mg/kg) and aspirin (30 mg/kg) beginning 2 days before operation in addition to the diet, and a third group received cod liver oil containing 1.8 grams of eicosapentaenoic acid daily 1 week before and for 6 weeks following operation. Serum cholesterol increased to similar levels in the 3 experimental groups and there were no detectable differences in bleeding parameters or platelet counts between the groups. Intimal thickness, which was assessed by microscopic evaluation of multiple segments of vein graft, increase from $4.5 \pm 0.2 \, \mu M$ at baseline (in a group of control dogs) $83 \pm 10 \, \mu M$ in dogs receiving the atherogenic diet alone. However, dogs receiving either the combination of aspirin and dipyridamole or those receiving cod liver oil both developed significantly smaller amounts of intimal hyperplasia. Of particular interest was the observation that vein grafts from dogs receiving cod liver oil had an average intimal thickness which was significantly less than that seen in the aspirin and dipyridamole group ($24 \pm 0.5 \, \mu M$ vs. $37 \pm 3 \, \mu M$; p<0.004). These findings demonstrate that dietary fish oil can inhibit intimal hyperplasia in vein grafts in hypercholesterolemic dogs and that the effect is significantly greater than that which is seen with anti-platelet agents. Although the mechanism responsible for the protective effects of dietary fish oil were not extensively evaluated, a reduction in plasma cholesterol levels does not appear to be involved. Since fibrous intimal hyperplasia is the primary cause of late bypass graft closure in humans, the results raise the possibility that dietary fish oil might have beneficial effects on graft patency in humans.

Fish oil and experimental atherosclerosis in rabbits

There have been several studies published recently in which the effects of dierary fish oil on atherogenesis in rabbits have been evaluated [13-17]. There have been important differences in the study design of these experiments including the methods used to stimulate atherosclerosis, the strain of rabbit used, the duration of the study and the type and amount of fish oil that was tested. The major findings of these studies are summarized in *Table II*. The anti-atherogenic effects of fish oil vary considerably with some studies suggesting enhanced lesion formation while others reported that there was either no significant effect or a reduction in atherosclerosis. The disparity in these results can be attributed to the differences in study design that were identified above. It is also important to note that the rabbit is a less than ideal model in which to evaluate the anti-atherogenic effects of dietary fish oil. Many of the studies used a high cholesterol diet to induce atherosclerosis. The level of cholesterol that was fed to rabbits tended to be extremely high in these studies compared to the amounts consumed by humans. The rabbit (unlike man) is extremely sensitive to dietary cholesterol and there are large differences in lipoprotein metabolism between rabbit and man. Finally, the

Table II. Studies of fish oil in rabbits

Investigators	Induction of athero-sclerosis	Fish oil	Duration of study	Effect on atherosclerosis
Thiery and Seidel.	1.5 % cholesterol diet	Ω-3 fatty acid* 2 ml/day	5 months	Increased in the aorta
Hearn *et al.*	2 % cholesterol and balloon injury	Ω-3 fatty acid 1 ml/day	6 weeks	Increased in the aorta ? diminished in the iliac artery
Rich *et al.*	Watanabe heritable hyperlipidemic rabbits	Ω-3 fatty acid 2.5 ml/day	12 months	No significant change
Bolton-Smith *et al.*	Serum sickness	Fish oil 20 g/kg	12 months	Decreased in the aorta
Zhu *et al.*	0.3 % cholesterol	1,2,3 ml Proto-chlo®	10 weeks	Decreased in the aorta with 2 and 3 ml doses

* Maxepa®

vascular lesions produced in the cholesterol-fed rabbit which are composed mostly of foam cells are quite dissimilar from the complicated lesions which developed in humans [18]. Thus, the relevance of the observations made in the cholesterol-fed rabbit in regards to human atherosclerosis is dubious.

Fish oil and coronary atherosclerosis in swine

Pigs are known to develop extensive atherosclerosis including coronary lesions which resemble those in humans in response to hypercholesterolemia. This process can be accelerated when there is arterial damage. In order to test the effects of dietary fish oil on coronary atherosclerosis in this model, Weiner *et al.* fed male Yorkshire pigs a 4 % cholesterol, high saturated fat diet over an 8 months period [19]. A subgroup of animals received 30 ml of cod liver oil (containing 12 % eicosapentaenoic acid) per day in addition to this diet. After 3 weeks, the pigs underwent balloon abrasion of the proximal left anterior descending coronary artery in order to accelerate the development of coronary lesions. After 8 months of experimental diet, the plasma cholesterol levels were 564 ± 203 mg/dL and 564 ± 106 mg/dL respectively in the control and fish oil groups. Neither lipoprotein fractions nor triglyceride levels differed between the study groups. Platelet fatty acid levels were unchanged from control levels in pigs receiving the high cholesterol diet alone. However, there were significant reductions in arachidonic acid and significant increases in eicosapentaenoic acid in platelets from fish oil fed animals. The effects of dietary fish oil on the development of coronary atherosclerosis are summarized in *Table III*. Significant reductions in all measures of coronary atherosclerosis were seen in the group receiving fish oil supplement. Of note is the fact that the protective effect was present in the left anterior descending coronary artery which underwent balloon abrasion as well as in right coronary and left circumflex coronary arteries which did not. These findings demonstrate that supplementation of an atherogenic diet with fish oil results in a marked reduction in coronary atherosclerosis in swine. The protective effects of fish oil occurred despite continued dietary uptake of large amounts of saturated fat and the presence of severe hyperlipidemia in this experimental model. Thus, it is likely that properties of dietary fish oil other than their effects on lipids and lipoproteins were responsible for their anti-atherogenic effects in this study. In this regard, plasma levels of thromboxane B2, a metabolic breakdown product of thromboxane A2, were reduced in the fish oil group but not in the control group during the course of the study. Since the release of thromboxane is an indicator of platelet activation, these findings are consistent with the hypothesis that the beneficial effects of fish oil on this study were the result of alterations in platelet function and a reduction in platelet-vessel wall interactions.

Table III. Coronary atherosclerosis in control and fish oil fed swine

	Control (n=11)	Oil fed (n=7)
Right coronary		
mean luminal encroachment (%)	53 ± 23	13 ± 14**
maximal luminal encroachment (%)	87	40**
lesion area (mm^2)	3.4 ±2.6	0.9 ± 2.0*
Left anterior descending coronary		
mean luminal encroachment (%)	44 ± 12	11 ± 16**
maximal luminal encroachment (%)	59	41**
lesion area (mm^2)	1.8 ±1.8	0.5 ± 1.3*
Left circumflex coronary		
mean luminal encroachment (%)	43 ± 16	5 ± 5**
maximal luminal encroachment (%)	62	11**
lesion area (mm^2)	1.4 ± 1.0	0.2 ± 0.1*

* $p < 0.05$; ** $p < 0.02$. (Adapted from reference [19]).

Effects of fish oil in non human primate models

Studies done in non human primates are extremely relevant to human disease. The digestive system, lipoprotein pattern and response to dietary cholesterol in these species are all very similar to those of humans. In addition, the atherosclerotic lesions that develop in response to a high cholesterol, high saturated fat diet are quite similar to those that are observed in human disease. Davis et al. studied the effects of dietary fish oil on the development of atherosclerosis in a group of adult male rhesus monkeys [20]. These animals received a 2 % cholesterol diet supplemented with varying amounts of experimental fats. Group 1 received 25 % of calories in the diet from coconut oil, a saturated fat which is known to be highly atherogenic. Group 2 received 25 % of calories from a combination of fish oil and coconut oil in a 1:1 ratio. Group 3 received 25 % of calories from fish oil and coconut oil in a 3:1 ratio. Plasma cholesterol levels rose to 875 mg/dL in group 1, and to 463 and 405 mg/dL in groups 2 and 3, respectively. HDL cholesterol was 49 mg/dL in group 1, 29 mg/dL in group 2, and 20 mg/dL in group 3. After 12 months of experimental diet, the animals were sacrificed and the amount of atherosclerosis was assessed in the aorta and in the carotid and femoral arteries. As shown in *Table IV*, the percent surface involvement with intimal lesions was significantly reduced in all of these arteries with the fish oil diet. In this study, fish oil inhibited the development of atherosclerosis in a non human primate model despite the presence of continued hypercholesterolemia. However, fish oil was associated with a reduction in serum cholesterol levels, suggesting that this mechanism may have been involved

Table IV. Surface involvement with intimal lesions in hypercholesterolemic monkeys

Group	Diet	Aorta (%)	Carotid (%)	Femoral (%)
I	Cholesterol and coconut oil	79 ± 5	49 ± 6	46 ± 6
II	Cholesterol and coconut oil/sigh oil (1:1)	48 ± 5*	22 ± 6	5 ± 1**
III	Cholesterol and coconut oil/fish oil (3:1)	36 ± 10**	3 ± 1**	3 ± 1**

* $p < 0.01$; ** $p < 0.001$. (Adapted from reference [20]).

in the anti-atherogenic effect. Interestingly, the high dose fish oil diet appeared to offer no greater protection than did the moderate fish oil diet in this experimental model.

Conclusions

In summary, dietary fish oil inhibits the development of atherosclerosis in most experimental animal models and there is evidence that intimal proliferation in vein grafts may also be reduced. Although changes in lipids and lipoprotein concentrations were associated with a reduction in atherosclerosis in some of the studies, they did not appear to be sufficient to account for the full extent of the anti-atherogenic effects of dietary fish oil. Platelet function was not extensively evaluated in these studies. However, the limited amount of information that is available suggests that alterations in platelet-vessel wall interactions may be involved in the anti-atherogenic effects of fish oil. Other factors including alterations in endothelium-derived relaxation factor (EDRF), growth factors and cytokines have not been studied during the development of experimental atherosclerosis. Based on their suspected role in atherogenesis, it is possible that changes in these pathways may account for at least some of the protective effects of dietary fish oil. Finally, it is important to note that there was little or no evidence of toxicity from dietary fish oil in the animal models used in these studies. However, this possibility was not extensively pursued in the studies that are described in this review and should be addressed by future studies.

References

1. Dyerberg J. Observations on populations in Greenland and Denmark. *In* : Barlow SM, Stanby M, eds. *Nutritional evaluation of long-term fatty acids in fish oil*. Orlando Academic Press, 1982; 245-261.

2. Kromhaut D, Bosschietger EB, Coulander CL. The inverse relationship between fish consumption and 20-year mortality from coronary heart disease. N Engl J Med 1985; 312 : 1205-1216.

3. Harris WS, Connor WE. The effects of salmon oil upon plasma lipids, lipoprotein and triglyceride clearance. Trans Assoc Am Phys 1980; 93 : 148-155.

4. Goodnight SH, Harris W, Connor WE. The effects of dietary Ω-3 fatty acids on platelet composition and function in man : a prospective, controlled study. Blood 1981; 58 : 880-885.

5. Knapp HR, Reilly IA, Alessandrini P *et al*. *In vivo* indexes of platelet and vascular function during fish-oil administration in patients with atherosclerosis. N Engl J Med 1986; 314 : 937-942.

6. von Schacky C, Fischer S, Weber PC. Long-term effects of dietary marine Ω-3 fatty acids upon plasma and cellular lipids, platelet function, and eicosanoid formation in humans. J Clin Invest 1985; 76 : 1626-1631.

7. Lee TH, Hoover RL, Williams JD *et al*. Effects of dietary enrichment with eicosapentoenoic and docosahexaenoic acids on *in vitro* neutrophil and monocyte leukotriene generation and neutrophil function. N Engl J Med 1985; 312 : 1217-1224.

8. Fox PL, DiCorleto PE. Fish oils inhibit endothelial cell production of platelet-derived growth factor-like protein. Science 1988; 214 : 453-456.

9. Shimokawa H, Lam JYT, Chesebro JH *et al*. Effects of dietary supplementation with cod liver oil on endothelium-dependent response in porcine coronary arteries. Circ 1987; 76 : 898-905.

10. Knapp HR, Fitzgerald GA. The antihypertensive effects of fish oil. A controlled study of polyunsaturated fatty acid supplements in essential hypertension. N Engl J Med 1989; 320 : 1037-1043.

11. Terano T, Hirai A, Hamazaki T *et al*. Effects of oral administration of highly purified eicosapentaenoic acid on platelet function, blood viscosity, and red cell deformability in healthy human subjects. Atherosclerosis 1983; 46 : 321-331.

12. Landymore RW, MacAulay M, Sheridan B *et al*. Comparison of cod liver oil and aspirin-dipyridamole for the prevention of intimal hyperplasia in autologous vein grafts. Ann Thorac Surg 1986; 41 : 54-57.

13. Thiery J, Seidel D. Fish oil feeding results in an enhancement of cholesterol-induced atherosclerosis in rabbits. Atherosclerosis 1987; 63 : 53-56.

14. Rich S, Miller JF, Charous S *et al*. Developement of atherosclerosis in genetically hyperlipidemic rabbits during chronic fish oil ingestion. Artherosclerosis 1989; 9 : 189-194.

15. Hearn JA, Sqoutas DS, Robinson KA *et al*. Marine lipid concentrate and atherosclerosis in the rabbit model. Atherosclerosis in the rabbit model. Atherosclerosis 1989; 75 : 39-47.

16. Bolton-Smith C, Gibney MJ, Gallagherg PJ *et al*. Effect of polyunsaturated fatty acid of the n-3 and n-6 series on lipid composition and cicosanoid synthesis of platelets and aorta and on immunological induction of atherosclerosis in rabbits. Atherosclerosis 1988; 72 : 29-35.

17. Zhu BQ. Smith DL, Siever RE *et al*. Inhibition of atherosclerosis by fish oil in cholesterol-fed rabbits. J Am Coll cardiol 1988; 12 : 1073-1078.

18. Stebbens WE. An appraisal of cholesterol feeding in experimental atherogenesis. Prog Cardiovasc Dis 1986; XXIX : 107-128.

19. Weiner BH, Ockene IS, Levine PH *et al*. Inhibition of atherosclerosis by cod liver oil in a hyperlipidemic swine model. N Engl J Med 1986; 89 : 941-846.

20. Davis HR, Bridenstine RT, Vesselinovitch D *et al*. Fish oil inhibits development of atherosclerosis in rhesus monkeys. Arteriosclerosis 1987; 7 : 441-449.

Fish oil and blood-vessel wall interactions. Eds P.M. Vanhoutte, Ph. Douste-Blazy.
John Libbey Eurotext, Paris © 1991, pp. 89-97.

9

Effect of chronic exposure to cod liver oil and Ω-3 unsaturated fatty acids on endothelium-dependent relaxations

C. Boulanger, V.B. Schini, H. Shimokawa, Th.F. Lüscher,
P.M. Vanhoutte

*Department of Research, University Hospital, CH-4031 Basel,
Switzerland, and Center for Experimental Therapeutics, Baylor College
of Medicine, Houston, TX 77030, USA.*

Abstract

The endothelium modulates the reactivity of the underlying vascular smooth muscle by releasing vasoactive substances. Thus, the endothelial cells produce prostacyclin and several endothelium-derived relaxing factors, one of which has been identified as nitric oxide. Endothelium-dependent relaxations are augmented in coronary arteries of pigs fed with cod liver oil or with its major component, eicosapentaenoic acid. This is due to an increased production of non-prostanoid relaxing factors from the intima of the blood vessels. An augmented release of relaxing factors also has been demonstrated with cultured endothelial cells chronically exposed to eicosapentaenoic acid. No increase in the production of endothelium-derived nitric oxide could be detected by activation of the soluble guanylate cyclase of cultured endothelial cells, suggesting that chronic exposure to eicosapentaenoic acid augments the release of the yet non-identified endothelium-derived relaxing factor which differs from nitric oxide. Dietary supplementation wich cod liver oil improves endothelium-dependent relaxations in hypercholesterolemic and atherosclerotic blood vessels : this effect could explain - in part - the beneficial effect of Ω-3 fatty acids on the occurence of cardiovascular diseases.

The endothelium modulates the reactivity of the smooth muscle by releasing different relaxing factors [1, 2]. Among these are (a) prostacyclin, produced during activation of the arachidonic acid cascade; (b) endothelium-derived relaxing factor (EDRF) recently identified as the radical nitric oxide [3, 5]; and (c) a non-identified endothelium-derived hyperpolarizing factor (EDHF) [6, 7] *(Figure 1)*. These three endothelial mediators induce-each to a certain extent - the relaxation of smooth muscle in a numerous variety of blood vessels including those of humans. This brief review will summarize the effect of chronic exposure to cod-liver oil or to Ω-3 unsaturated fatty acid on endothelium-dependent relaxations and the production of non-prostanoid relaxing factors by endothelial cells.

Relaxing factors produced by the endothelium

A non-prostanoid relaxing factor [3] released by the vascular endothelium shares pharmacological properties with the radical nitric oxide [8, 9]. In many bioassay studies, the release of nitric oxide from endothelial cells and from the endothelium of isolated blood vessels accounts for the relaxing activity of the perfusate [4, 10]. As endothelium-derived relaxing factor, nitric oxide induces relaxation of vascular smooth muscle by activating soluble guanylate cyclase and this effect is inhibited by methylene blue; nitric oxide is also scavenged by hemoglobin and inactivated by superoxide anions. Nitric oxide is synthetized in endothelial cells from the amino acid L-arginine [11]. The enzymatic conversion of L-arginine to nitric oxide is inhibited by an L-N^G monomethyl analog of the amino acid [12]. *In vivo* blockade of nitric oxide synthesis leads to an increase in blood pressure [5]. However, the release of nitric oxide from the endothelium as a single radical is still controversial : for example, nitric oxide might bind a carrier, the amino acid cysteine, and be released as nitrocysteine [13].

In addition to nitric oxide, endothelial cells release another relaxing factor, called endothelium-derived hyperpolarizing factor (EDHF). In canine arteries, the relaxation and the hyperpolarization of the smooth muscle that EDHF induces are sensitive to ouabain [6]. Endothelium-derived nitric oxide does not modify the membrane potential of arterial smooth muscle and its effect is insensitive to ouabain [14]. The relaxing factor that differs from nitric oxide has a more pronounced effect in blood vessels of small diameter [15]. Endothelium-derived hyperpolarizing factor could initiate the endothelium-dependent relaxations; alternatively, it could increase the action of nitric oxide on smooth muscle.

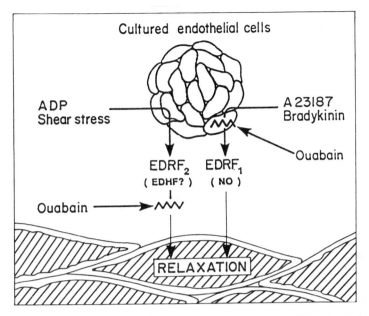

Figure 1. Schematic representation of the release of at least two different relaxing factors from cultured porcine endothelial cells. Bradykinin and the calcium ionophore A23187 release by a ouabain-sensitive mechanism, a relaxing factor which induces relaxation of canine coronary smooth muscle as nitric oxide does. The effect of the relaxing factor released by adenosine diphosphate (ADP) and under shear stress conditions, is impaired in the presence of ouabain; this relaxing factor possesses similar properties to endothelium-derived hyperpolarizing factor (EDHF). (From reference [16], by permission).

The release of prostanoids and non-prostanoids relaxing factors can be observed from cultured endothelial cells. The relaxing activity of the superfusate of cultured endothelial cells grown on microcarrier beads and packed into a chromatographic column is assessed usually using a ring of blood vessel without endothelium as detector. The influence of vasoactive prostanoids can be ruled out by performing the experiments in the presence of an inhibitor of cyclooxygenase. The release of non-prostanoid relaxing factors can be observed both under basal conditions and upon stimulation with bradykinin, adenosine diphosphate or the calcium inophore A23187 *(Figure 1)* [16]. Under these bioassay conditions, cultured endothelial cells from the porcine aorta release two relaxing factors, one being most likely nitric oxide. These two factors can be differentiated with ouabain. Bradykinin and the calcium inophore A23187 release a relaxing factor which is similar to nitric oxide; its action is unopposed by ouabain. Another relaxing factor is released spontaneously or upon stimulation with adenosine diphosphate : its effect on vascular smooth muscle is inhibited by the cardenolide [16]. Methylene blue and hemoglobin inhibit the relaxation induced by exogenous nitric oxide and that induced by bradykinin; however, they only partially impair that mediated by adenosine diphosphate.

Effect of cod-liver oil and Ω-3 unsaturated fatty acids on endothelium-dependent relaxations

Dietary supplementation with cod-liver oil increases the endothelium-dependent relaxations of porcine coronary arteries induced by aggregating platelets, bradykinin, thrombin and products of platelet aggregation, but not those mediated by the calcium ionophore A23187 *(Figure 2)* [17]. This indicates that the basic process leading to the release of endothelium-derived relaxing factor(s) is not affected. The same effect induced by cod-fish oil can be reproduced in large coronary arteries and coronary microvessels of pigs fed with eicosapentaenoic acid, the major component of marine oils [18, 19] *(Figure 3)*. Bioassay experiments demonstrate that bradykinin releases relaxing factors to a greater extent from the intima of blood vessels obtained from animals treated with the Ω-3 unsaturated fatty acid [18].

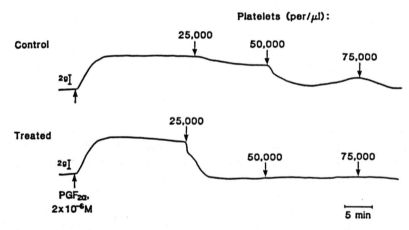

Figure 2. Effect of chronic intake of cod-liver oil on the response of porcine coronary arteries to aggregating platelets. The porcine coronary arteries with endothelium were first contracted with prostaglandin F2alpha (PGF2α) before the addition of increasing number of platelets to the organ chambers. Please note the higher relaxation induced by the platelets in the blood vessels of animals fed with cod liver oil. (From reference [17], by permission).

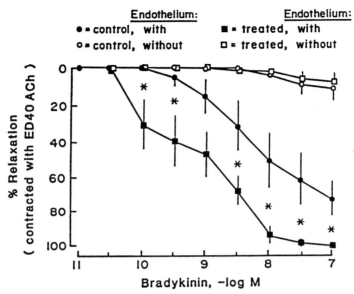

Figure 3. Effect of dietary supplementation of pigs with Ω3-unsaturated fatty acids on the response of porcine coronary resistance microvessels with endothelium to bradykinin. Experiments were realized in the presence of indomethacin to inhibit the production of vasoactive prostanoids. (From Reference [18], with permission).

In order to delineate which of the endothelial mediators was involved in the response induced by chronic exposure to Ω-3 fatty acids, cultured endothelial cells were exposed for several days to eicosapentaenoic acid (2.5×10^{-5} M). The release of relaxing substances from cultured endothelial cells was determined under bioassay conditions [20]. Chronic exposure to eicosapentaenoic acid augmented the relaxations mediated by bradykinin and to a larger extent those induced by adenosine diphosphate, but it did not affect those evoked by the calcium ionophore A23187 *(Figure 4)*. The production of endothelium-derived nitric oxide by cultured endothelial cells can be detected by the activation of the soluble guanylate cyclase and further accumulation of cyclic GMP in the endothelial cells. Stimulation of cultured endothelial cells by exogenous nitric oxide and by agents releasing relaxing factor(s) induced a rapid and transient increase of the intracellular level of cyclic GMP which was inhibited by methylene blue and by L-N^{G} monomethyl arginine [21]. No difference in cyclic GMP accumulation was found in cells exposed to eicosapentaenoic acid when compared to control *(Figure 5)*. These results suggest that chronic exposure to eicosapentaenoic acid does not improve the production of endothelium-derived nitric oxide but favors the release of another non-prostanoid relaxing factor [20].

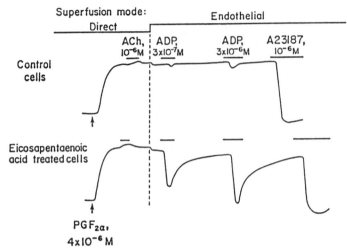

Figure 4. Effect of chronic exposure of cultured endothelial cells to eicosapentaenoic acid on the production of relaxing factors under bioassay condition. The relaxing activity of a perfusate of control or eicosapentaenoic-acid treated endothelial cells was assessed with a canine coronary artery rings (bioassay rings) without endothelium. The bioassay ring were contracted under a column of beads without cells with prostaglandin F2 α, and then moved under a column of microcarrier beads coated with cultured endothelial cells to detect the release of relaxing factors upon stimulation with adenosine diphosphate (ADP) or the calcium ionophore A23187. The relaxing activity of the perfusate from cells exposed to eicopentaenoic acid was higher than that observed with control cultures. (From reference [20], by permission).

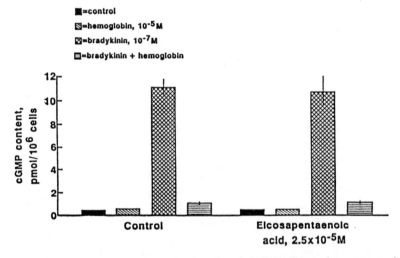

Figure 5. Effect of chronic exposure of cultured endothelial cells to eicosapentaenoic acid on the production of cyclic GMP upon stimulation with bradykinin. The accumulation of cyclic GMP was determined after 1 min stimulation, in the presence of indomethracin and isobutylmethyl xanthine. Cyclic GMP was determined with a radioimmunoassay and expressed as pmol/million cells. (From reference [20], by permission).

Ω-3 unsaturated fatty acids and cardiovascular disease

Injury of dysfunction of the endothelial layer plays a major role in the pathogenesis of atherosclerosis [22]. The endothelium-dependent responses to aggregating platelets and related vasoactive substances (serotonin and adenosine diphosphate) are impaired in coronary arteries of hypercholesterolemic pigs or in those with regenerated endothelium [23, 24]. These responses are blunted even further in atherosclerotic blood vessels. This impaired relaxation is probably due to a reduced release of endothelium-derived relaxing factors [23]. The interactions between platelets and atherosclerotic blood vessels would favor platelet aggregation and platelets-induced contractions of vascular smooth muscle; this could lead to vasospasm and thrombosis. Dietary supplementation with Ω-3 unsaturated fatty acids may delay the impairment of endothelium-dependent relaxations in hypercholesterolemia and in atherosclerosis, partly by improving the release of endothelium-derived relaxing factors [25, 26] *(Figure 6)*.

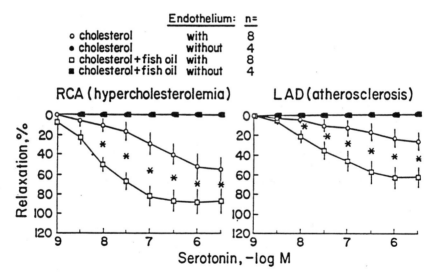

Figure 6. Effect of dietary supplementation with cod liver oil of pigs fed with a regime high in cholesterol on endothelium-dependent relaxation evoked by serotonin in coronary arteries. Compare the response of the right coronary artery (RCA) to that of the left descending coronary artery (LAD), with has been previously denuded by the means of a balloon catheter. Experiments were performed in the presence of indomethacin and ketanserin. (From Reference [25], with permision).

References

1. Furchgott RF, Vanhoutte PM. Endothelium-derived relaxing and contracting factors. The Faseb J 1989; 3 : 2007-2018.

2. Lüscher TF, Vanhoutte PM. The endothelium : Modulator of cardiovascular function. CRC Press, Boca Raton, 1990 (in press).

3. Furchgott RF, Zawadzki JV. The obligatory role of endothelial cells in the relaxation of arterial smooth muscle by acetylcholine. Nature 1980; 299 : 373-376.

4. Palmer RMJ, Ferrige AG, Moncada S. Nitric oxide release accounts for the biological activity of endothelium-derived relaxing factor. Nature 1987; 327 : 524-526.

5. Rees DD, Palmer RMJ, Moncada S. The role of endothelium-derived nitric oxide in the regulation of blood pressure. Proc Natl Acad Sci USA 1989; 86 : 3375-3378.

6. Feletou M, Vanhoutte PM. Endothelium-dependent hyperpolarization of canine coronary smooth muscle. Br J Pharmacol 1988; 93 : 515-524.

7. Bény J-L, Brunet PC. Electrophysiological and mechanical effects of substance P and acetylcholine on rabbit aorta. J Physiol 1988; 398 : 277-289.

8. Furchgott RF, Khan MT, Jothianandan D *et al*. Evidence that the endothelium-derived relaxing factor of rabbit aorta is nitric oxide. *In : Vascular Neuroeffector Mechanisms* Vol 10, Bevan JA, Majewski H, Maxwell RA and Story DF, eds, IRL Press, Oxford, England, 1988; pp 77-84.

9. Ignarro LJ, Byrns RE, Wood KS. Biochemical and pharmacological properties of endothelium-derived relaxing factor and its similarity to nitric oxide radical. *In : Vasodilatation : Vascular Smooth Muscle, Peptides, Autonomic Nerves and Endothelium*. PM Vanhoutte, ed, Raven Press, New York, NY, 1988; pp 427-436.

10. Amezcua JL, Dusting GJ, Palmer RMJ *et al*. Acetylcholine induces vasodilatation in the rabbit isolated heart through the release of nitric oxide, the endogenous nitrovasodilator. Br J Pharmacol 1988; 95 : 830-834.

11. Palmer RMJ, Ashton DS, Moncada S. Vascular endothelial cells synthesize nitric oxide from L-arginine. Nature 1988; 333 : 664-666.

12. Rees DD, Palmer RMJ, Hodson HF *et al*. A specific inhibitor of nitric oxide formation from L-arginine attenuates endothelium-dependent relaxation. Br J Pharmacol 1989; 96 : 418-424.

13. Myers PR, Guerra R Jr, Bates JN *et al*. Studies on the properties of endothelium-derived relaxing factor (EDRF), nitric oxide, and nitrosothiols : Similarities between EDRF and S-nitroso-L-cysteine (cysNO) (Abstract). J Vasc Med Biol 1989; 1/2 : 106.

14. Komori K, Lorenz RR, Vanhoutte PM. Nitric oxide, acetylcholine, and electrical and mechanical properties of canine arterial smooth muscle. Am J Physiol 1988; 255 : H207-H212.

15. Hoeffner U, Boulanger C, Vanhoutte PM. Proximal and distal coronary arteries respond differently to basal EDRF but not to NO. Am J Physiol 1989; 256 : H828-H831.

16. Boulanger C, Hendrickson H, Lorenz RR *et al*. Release of different relaxing factors by cultured porcine endothelial cells. Circ Res 1989; 64 : 1070-1078.

17. Shimokawa H, Lam JYT, Chesebro JH *et al*. Effects of dietary supplementation with cod-liver oil on endothelium-dependent responses in porcine coronary arteries. Circulation 1987; 76 : 898-905.

18. Shimokawa H, Aarhus LL, Vanhoutte PM. Dietary Ω-3 polyunsaturated fatty acids augment endothelium-dependent relaxation to bradykinin in porcine coronary microvessels. Br J Pharmacol 1989; 95 : 1191-1196.

19. Shimokawa H, Vanhoutte PM. Dietary Ω-3 fatty acids and endothelium-dependent relaxations in porcine coronary arteries. Am J Physiol 1989; 256 : H968-H973.

20. Boulanger C, Schini VB, Hendrickson H *et al*. Chronic exposure of cultured endothelial cells to eicosapentaenoic acid potentiates the release of endothelium-derived relaxing factor(s). Br J Pharmacol 1990; 99 : 176-180.

21. Boulanger C, Schini VB, Vanhoutte PM. Production of cyclic GMP by bradykinin, adenosine diphosphate, the calcium ionophore A23187 and nitric oxide in cultured porcine aortic endothelial cells. Faseb J 1989; 3 : A533.

22. Ross R. The pathogenesis of atherosclerosis- An update. New Engl J Med 1986; 314 : 488-500.

23. Shimokawa H, Vanhoutte PM. Impaired endothelium-dependent relaxation to aggregating platelets and related vasoactive substances in porcine coronary arteries in hypercholesterolemia and atherosclerosis. Circ Res 1989; 64 : 900-914.

24. Shimokawa H, Aarhus LL, Vanhoutte PM. Porcine coronary arteries with regenerated endothelium have a reduced endothelium-dependent responsiveness to aggregating platelets and serotonin. Circ Res 1987; 61 : 256-270.

25. Shimokawa H, Vanhoutte PM. Dietary cod-liver oil improves endothelium-dependent responses in hypercholesterolemic and atherosclerotic porcine coronary arteries. Circulation 1988; 78 : 1421-1430.

26. Shimokawa H, Vanhoutte PM. Hypercholesterolemia causes generalized impairment of endothelium-dependent relaxation to aggregating platelets in porcine arteries. J Amer Coll Cardiol 1989; in press.

Fish oil and blood-vessel wall interactions. Eds P.M. Vanhoutte, Ph. Douste-Blazy.
John Libbey Eurotext, Paris © 1991, pp. 99-107.

10

Ω-3 fatty acids and microcirculation

G. Bruckner

Department of Clinical Sciences, University of Kentucky, USA.

Abstract

Three studies were conducted to determine the effects of different fats on blood flow in peripheral blood vessels, the type of dietary fat which has the greatest effect on peripheral blood flow and the effect of supplemented dietary vitamin E on the microcirculation. In normolipidemic adults, dietary fats rich in Ω-3 vs. Ω-9 fatty acid significantly increased nailfold capillary blood cell velocities. Hyperlipidemic adults responded to fats rich in Ω-3 and Ω-6 fatty acids with increases in capillary blood cell velocities. These changes in hyperlipidemia were persistent after a one month washout period. Geriatric normolipidemic individuals only showed significant increased blood flow velocities following Ω-3 fatty acid and vitamin E supplementation. This data suggests that Ω-3 and Ω-6 fatty acids, with adequate antioxidants, most likely increase peripheral capillary blood flow by altering vascular tone and blood viscosity. Furthermore, Ω-3 fatty acids without adequate antioxidant present may be detrimental with regard to peripheral capillary flow.

Introduction

Cardiovascular disease is one of the most significant dietary related health problems in the United States of America [1]. During the past decade a great deal of progress has been made toward defining the role of dietary fats and hypercholesterolemia in the pathogenesis of arteriosclerosis [2] and this, along with more public nutrition education, may be related to the observed steady decline in morbidity and mortality from cardiovascular disease [3]. The etiology of cardiovascular disease is multifaceted and although

99

many findings support the involvement of dietary fat and cholesterol in atherogenesis [1, 4], the mechanisms involved are not clearly understood. For example, it is known that different fatty acid isomers, Ω-3 vs. Ω-6 20 carbon fatty acids, can elicit completely different vascular responses as evidenced by the Greenland Eskimo studies and subsequent reports by Dyerberg and Bang [5] and others [6-9]. Recent work by Grundy [10] also suggests that various monounsaturated fatty acids can have different cholesterol-lowering effects. Therefore, it is evident that a number of factors in addition to serum cholesterol are involved in the etiology of cardiovascular disease, e.g. blood flow, platelet endothelial interaction, lipid hydroperoxides, etc. Changes in capillary blood flow have been noted in subjects with atherosclerotic disease [11], however it is not clear whether these changes contribute to the etiology of the disease or are the consequence of the disease process. Changes in blood flow and platelet-endothelial cell interactions have been implicated to directly influence atherogenesis [12]. We postulate that the interactions of circulating lipids with endothelial surfaces depend in part on the rate of blood flow. The constant exposure of the endothelium to various blood components, including prooxidants such as fatty acid peroxides or oxidized derivatives of cholesterol, may damage or alter a number of endothelial cell functions, e.g. synthesis of antiaggregatory vasodilators (prostacyclin), endothelial cell permeability and/or platelet endothelial cell adhesion. It is possible that these lipids, particularly the oxidized forms, along with the products of cellular metabolism, may elicit greater cellular damage in slower flowing vessels. This may be due to prolonged contact with these surfaces, resulting in an increased chance for initiation of lesion development. Therefore, it is important to better understand the effects of different fatty acids on blood flow. Moreover, due to the differing susceptibility of various fatty acids to oxidative reactions it is important to determine the degree to which these fatty acids are oxidized and their effects on events associated with microcirculatory changes and atherogenesis. Our ongoing studies are designed to help us better understand 1) the effects of different fats on blood flow in peripheral blood vessels and the underlying mechanism involved, 2) the amount and type of dietary fatty acid which has the greatest effect on peripheral blood flow, and 3) the effect of the dietary antioxidant vitamin E on the microcirculation.

Methods and results

Three studies have been conducted to assess the effects of Ω-3 fatty acid supplementation on microcirculatory changes.

Study number 1

Twelve normolipidemic male subjects (cholesterol <220, triglycerides <250) were recruited for the study aged 18-40. The study was a parallel design with no crossover. Subjects were randomly allocated to fish oil (Ω-3 fatty acid*) or olive oil supplemented groups at 1.5 g oil/10, kg Bwt/day. All capsules contained 1 I.U. vitamin E/g oil. Nailfold capillary blood cell velocities were measured before and after 3 weeks of supplementation as well as biochemical lipid parameters (cholesterol, triglycerides, and high density lipoproteins). These results and the microcirculatory methodologies have been previously published [7] and are depicted in *Figure 1*. Capillary blood cell velocity was significantly increased by fish vs. olive oil supplementation. No washout measurements were made.

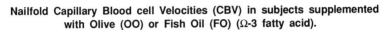

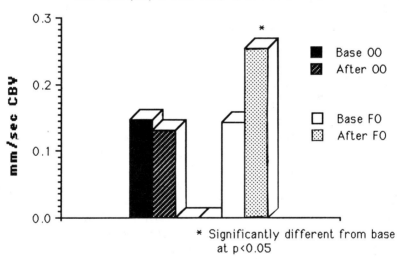

Figure 1. Changes in nailfold capillary blood cell velocities before and after three weeks supplementation with olive or fish oil at 1.5 g oil/kg Bwt/day.

Study number 2.

Thirty-two hyperlipidemic (cholesterol 220 mg/dl and triglycerides 250 mg/dl) male subjects aged 18-55 were recruited and randomly allocated

---

(*) Maxepa®.

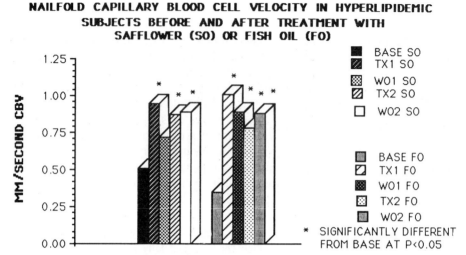

Figure 2. Changes in nailfold capillary blood cell velocities before (base), after two months supplementation with fish or safflower oil (TX₁), following one month washout prior to next treatment regimen (WO₁), and after treatment two (TX₂) or washout 2 (WO₂).

to four treatment groups; fish oil and oat bran, fish oil (Ω-3 fatty acid) and wheat bran, safflower oil and oat branch or safflower oil and wheat bran. Oils were supplemented at 1.5 g oil/10 kg Bwt/day and bran at approximately 10 g total fiber/subject/day. The experimental design was a crossover design balanced for residual effects. Each subject therefore received each treatment combination over the course of one year. Baseline or washout measurements for capillary blood cell velocity were determined on all subjects prior to and after two months of treatment. All subjects discontinued supplements for one month washout before starting the next regimen. As shown in *Figure 2,* capillary blood cell velocity was increased significantly by fish oil and safflower oil supplementation over baseline. Fiber did not contribute to capillary blood cell velocity changes. Capillary blood cell velocity never returned to the original baseline values after either fish or safflower oil intervention, although serum fatty acids returned to normal values after a one month washout period (data not shown).

Study number 3

Forty normolipidemic (cholesterol <220, triglycerides <250) male geriatric subjects (55-70) were recruited through the Sanders-Brown Aging Center at the University of Kentucky. They were randomly allocated to 4 groups as follows : Purified fish oil product containing approximately 50 % Ω-3 fatty

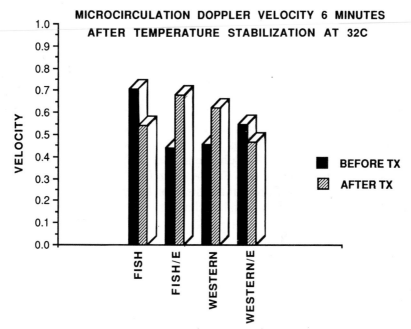

Figure 3. Changes in subdermal blood flow velocity as measured by laser doppler in Hz units before and after 4 weeks supplementation with the various oils with or without 800 I.U. Vit E/day. All oils supplemented at 1.5 g/10 kg Bwt/day. Only fish/E after TX is significantly different from before TX at p .05.

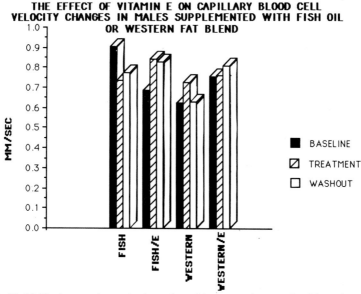

Figure 4. Nailfold changes in geriatric male subjects supplemented with various oils for 4 weeks (treatment) at 1.5 g/10 kg Bwt/day with or without 800 I.U./day vitamin E. Washout measurements were conducted 4 months after supplements were discontinued.

103

acid with or without vitamin E, and Western diet fat blend with or without vitamin E (a mixture of lard, tallow and corn oil to mimic average daily fat intake in US population). All oils were given at 1.5 g/10 kg Bwt/day. Vitamin E supplemented at 800 I.U./day. Laser doppler flow and capillary blood cell velocity measurements were made before and after two months of supplementation and followings two months washout. The fish oil with vitamin E increased velocity of subdermal and CBV as measured by laser doppler and videomicroscopy (see *Figures 3 and 4*). However, the fish treatment alone decreased CBV from that noted for baseline and the other treatments which did not result in notable changes.

Blood pressure, serum lipids and blood viscosity were measured as previously reported [7] in all three studies.

Discussion

Ω-3 fatty acid related factors which may affect peripheral microcirculation are blood pressure, blood viscosity and vascular tone *(Figure 5)*. Systemic

VASCULAR MECHANISMS ALTERED BY N3 FATTY ACIDS

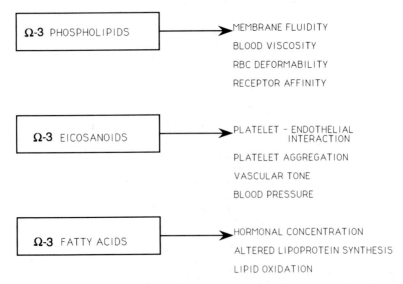

Figure 5. Ω-3 fatty acid may alter vascular responses via incorporation into phospholipids and/or subsequent release as eicosanoid precursors or perhaps directly by alteration of hormonal, lipoprotein or lipid peroxide synthesis.

blood pressure was measured in all these studies with no significant changes noted prior to or after oil supplementation. Additionally one would expect increased capillary blood cell velocity to be associated with increased blood pressure changes however, other investigators have demonstrated a decrease in systemic pressure following fish oil intervention [13].

Blood viscosity was measured in these studies using a capillary viscometer. There were no significant changes noted for plasma or whole blood using this method to determine blood viscosity, however, these measurements may differ from the results of others using a cone viscometer [14]. Both methods should be employed in future studies to help define these differences.

Our studies suggest that in humans, increased capillary blood cell velocity is most likely due to changes in precapillary vascular tone, i.e. vasodilatation, however, it is not clear what events bring about these changes *(Figure 6)*.

Changes in vascular tone may be altered by eicosanoid ratios (TXA_3/PGI_3; TXA_2/PGI_2) [15, 16], hormone concentrations, membrane structural changes and/or receptor agonist binding.

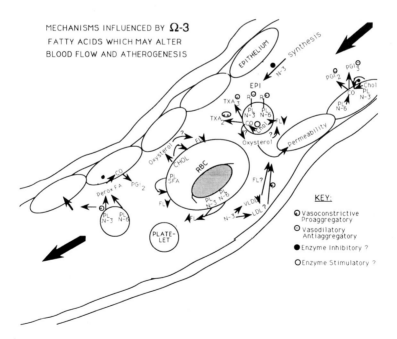

Figure 6. Ω-3 fatty acid may alter blood flow and atherogenesis by mechanism favoring the promotion of antiaggregatory and vasodilatory eicosanoids or altering membrane fluidity. These events may be altered by membrane viscosity and changes in circulating lipids and lipoproteins.

105

As depicted in *Figure 6,* we hypothesize that events which alter lipid per-oxidation, eicosanoid production or membrane fluidity may alter vascular hemodynamics through a number of mechanisms. For example, if cholesterol is incorporated into platelet membranes, the increased production of vaso-constrictive eicosanoids (TXA_2) might be stimulated. Furthermore, cholesterol may decrease fluidity of the platelet and RBC membrane. We also speculate that cholesterol oxides may be produced from oxygenase ac-tivities which could lead to further vascular damage due to increased en-dothelial cell permeability. Ω-3 fatty acids may alter these events by favoring the production of vasodilatory eicosanoids and decreasing membrane fluidity, provided that these highly oxidizable lipids are protected by adequate an-tioxidants.

It is also possible that subtle insignificant individual changes in each of the three variables i.e. blood pressure, blood viscosity and vascular tone when combined may contribute to the significant changes which we have noted as increased capillary blood cell velocity after intervention with dietary Ω-3 or Ω-6 fatty acids. Additionally as suggested by the results of study number 3, the antioxidant status of the individual may determine if the addition of dietary unsaturated fatty acids is beneficial or detrimental to changes in pe-ripheral microcirculation.

References

1. Surgeon General's Report on Nutrition and Health, US Department of Health and Human Services, 1988; DHHS No. 88-5021.
2. St Clair RW. Pathogenesis of the Atherosclerotic Lesion : Current Concepts of Cellular and Biochemical Events. Recent Advances in Arterial Diseases : Atherosclerosis, Hyper-tension, and Vasospasm. New York : Alan R. Liss, Inc 1986; 1-29.
3. Higgins MW, Lenfant CJM. Trends in Cornary Heart Disease. Arch Mal Cœur 1989; Vol 7, 82 : 2041-7.
4. Sexton RC, Rudney H. Regulation of Cholesterol Biosynthesis. Ann Review Nutr 1986; 6 : 245-272.
5. Dyerberg J., Bang HO. Lipid Metabolism, Atherogenesis, and Haemostasis in Eskimos : The Role of the Prostaglandin-3 Family. Haemostasis 1979; 8 (3-5) : 227-33.
6. Kinsella, JE. Seafoods and Fish Oils in Human Health and Disease. New York : Marcel Dekker, Inc 1987.
7. Bruckner G, Webb P, Greenwell L *et al.* Fish Oil Increases Peripheral Capillary Blood Cell Velocity in Humans. Atherosclerosis 1987; 66 : 237-45.
8. Lands VEM. Fish and Human Health. Orlando : Academic Press 1986.
9. Webb P, Bond V, Kotchen T *et al.* Polyunsaturated Fatty Acids and Eicosanoids. Biloxi : Am Oil Chemists Soc 1987; 329-333.

10. Grundy SM. Comparison of Monounsaturated Fatty Acids and Carbohydrates for Lowering Plasma Cholesterol. NEJM 1986; 314 : 745-48.

11. Schwartz RW, Freedman AM, Richardson DR, *et al.* Capillary Blood Flow : Videodensitometry in the Atherosclerotic Patient. J Vas Surg 1984; 1 : 800-808.

12. Ross R, Glomset J. The Pathogenesis of Atherosclerosis. NEJM 1976; 295 : 369-376.

13. Knapp HR. Ω-3 fatty acids, Endogenous Prostaglandins, and Blood Pressure Regulation in Humans. Nutr Rev 1989; 47 : 301-313.

14. Kobayashi S, Hirai A, Terano T *et al.* Reduction in Blood Viscosity by Eicosapentaenoic Acid. Lancet 1981; 2 : 197.

15. Fisher S, Weber PG. Prostaglandin I3 is Formed *in vivo* in Man after Dietary Eicosapentanaeonoic Acid. Nature 1984; 307 : 165-67.

16. Juan H, Sametz. Vascular Reactivity and High Deietary Eicosapentaenoic Acid. Naunyn-Schmiedeberg's Pharmacol 1986; 24 : 631-639.

Fish oil and blood-vessel wall interactions. Eds P.M. Vanhoutte, Ph. Douste-Blazy.
John Libbey Eurotext, Paris © 1991, pp. 109-116.

11

Coronary heart disease and Ω-3 : epidemiological aspects.

H.O. Bang

Huidegardsparken 43, 02800 Lyngby, Danemark.

Abstract

Two decades an explanation was sought for the infrequency of thrombotic diseases, especially ischaemic heart disease in Greenland Eskimos.
In many of the settlements in Greenland, ischaemic heart disease is almost never observed. In the whole of Greenland, including the cities, the frequency of ischaemic heart disease is one tenth of that in Denmark. We carried out four expeditions to the Umanaq district in the north-western part of Greenland, some 500 km north of the polar circle. We measured the blood lipids in 130 Greenlanders aged more than 40 years. We found the total cholesterol level a little lower than that of Danish controls, the triglycerides much lower, the LDL level a little and the VLDL level much lower than the controls. The HDL in males was higher than in the controls. The fatty acid pattern in ester-bound with cholesterol, triglycerides, and phospholipids was very different from that of Danes, with low concentration of the Ω-6 fatty acid and much higher level of the Ω-3 fatty acid, predominantly C 20 : 5 Ω-3 EPA and C 22 : 6 Ω-3 DHA. The blood lipids of Greenlanders living in Denmark was identical with that of Danes. Consequently, the peculiar pattern of fatty acid in the Eskimos must be of extern, probably nutritional origin. Examinations of the diets of the Eskimos, carried out in two further expeditions, with 248 food specimens, showed a similar pattern of fatty acids as that found in the blood.
We found in laboratory studies that the Eskimos can «use» EPA as precursor of platelet active prostanoids instead of arachidonic acid which is the precursor of these prostanoids in the Western world. Furthermore, we found the balance between the platelet proaggregatory thromboxane and the antiaggregatory prostacyclin shifted in an antiaggregatory direction.

Experiments in our laboratory and examinations during another expedition to Greenland showed that the platelet aggregability was reduced and the bleeding time increased in the Eskimos. We concluded that this was the explanation of the rarity of thrombotic diseases in Greenland. Japanese researchers examined in a similar way the blood lipids and platelet behavior in Japanese fishermen as compared with farmers with the same results as ours.

Many studies in animals and several in humans have confirmed our results and widened our knowledge of the favorable effects of Ω-3 fatty acids of marine origin. Lately clinical observations have been published showing that supplementation of EPA and DHA to some degree prohibits restenosis after coronary angioplasty and results in fewer new cases of coronary thrombosis in patients who have survived their first attack of this disease.

It has long been noticed that thrombotic diseases, especially ischaemic heart disease is infrequent in Greenland Eskimos. In the small settlements in the far North ischaemic heart disease is very seldom observed. In the whole of Greenland with the cities the prevalence of ischaemic heart disease is about one tenth of that of Danes [1].

In the late sixties, I throught of trying to find the cause of this peculiar pattern of disease. My collegue Dr. Jørn Dyerberg joined me.

We carried out together four expeditions to the northwestern part of Greenland, the Umanaq district, 500 km north of the Polar Circle, with some 2 500 inhabitants. In this part of Greenland the original Eskimo lifestyle, almost exclusively as hunters and/or fishermen, still exists. Especially, western food is of rather little importance. The nutrition consists rather exclusively of meat from the arctic animals whale and seal, and fish. We calculated that each Greenlander, from baby to elderly, consumed averagely about 400 g seal meat a day [2].

During the first expedition we took 130 blood specimens in fasting people aged 40 years and above and measured the serum lipid patterns including quantitation of the lipopoteins by means of electrophoresis. We found lower levels of serum cholesterol and low density lipoprotein, much lower levels of serum triglycerides and very low density lipoprotein and – in the males – higher levels of high density lipoprotein as compared with Danish controls [3] (*Table I*).

Furthermore, we measured with gas liquid chromatography the plasma fatty acids in ester-bound with cholesterol, triglycerides, and phospholipids. We found a fatty acid pattern very different from that of Danes. The concentrations of the fatty acids of the C : 18 series and the Ω-6 and Ω-9 families were much lower than in Danes. But the level of the long-chained fatty acids with 20 and 22 carbon atoms and belonging to the Ω-3 family was much higher in the Eskimos, with at factor 4 to 14 as compared with Danish

Table I. Plasma lipids and fatty acid patterns in
Greenland Eskimos and Danish controls [3, 4].

	Eskimos	Danes
S. cholesterol g/l	2.28	2.80
S. triglycerides g/l	0.51	1.19
S. LDL g/l	4.42	5.21
S. VLDL g/l	0.46	1.45
S.C 18 : 2 Ω-6 as cholesterol ester % of total fatty acid	20.3	51.0
S.C 20 : 5 Ω-3 as cholesterol ester % of total fatty acid	15.8	0.9
S.C 22 : 6 Ω-3 as cholesterol ester % of total fatty acid	1.0	0.4

controls [4]. This observation was new. So thorough an examination of the blood lipids had never before been carried out in an ethnic population.

In order to find out if this peculiar Eskimo blood lipid pattern was not of genetic, racial origin, we measured the blood lipids in Eskimos living in Denmark and with a lifestyle similar to other Danes and found no difference between these Eskimos and Danes.

Consequently, the peculiar blood lipid patterns of the Eskimos must be of exogen, probably of nutritional origin. During two further expeditions to the same part of Greenland we collected 227 specimens of food, using the Double Portion Technique by Ancel Keys [5]. We examined the composition of the Eskimo diet and found it very rich in proteins, rather poor in carbohydrates, and similar in the fat content as Danish food. The fatty acid pattern in the dietary fats was rather similar to that of the blood lipids in the Eskimos [2].

At that time, in the middle of the seventies, the blood platelet active prostanoids thromboxane (TXA 2) and prostacyclin (PGI 2) had been described. Both have arachidonic acid (C 20 : 4 Ω-6) as precursor. As this fatty acid is rather scarce in the Eskimos' blood (from one eighth to one third as compared with Danish controls) and another fatty acid with 20 carbon atoms eicosapentaenoic acid (EPA) is rather rich, it was natural to ask if the Eskimos could «use» EPA as precursor of platelet active prostanoids, and if this be so, if the balance between the platelet pro-aggregatory and vasoconstrictive thromboxane and the anti-aggregatory and vasodilatory prostacyclin is shifted towards a dominant role of prostacyclin. Test tube experiments we carried out showed this to be the case. With EPA as precursor the production of thromboxane TXA 2 is reduced and an inactive thromboxane TXA 3 is formed. The production of prostacyclin PGI 2 is enhanced and another prostacyclin PGI 3 which is as active as PGI 2 is produced [6, 7, 8].

Consequently, with EPA as precursor the platelet active prostanoids are less platelet aggregatory and hence less thrombogenic.

We would at that time like to test if Eskimo food had the property as we though. However it was not possible in Denmark to get hold of seal or whale meat, but cod liver oil contains about 20 % EPA. So we gave Danish volunteers big doses of this fish oil, and we could observe changes toward a similar blood lipid pattern as that of the Eskimos, and furthermore a decreased platelet aggregability and increased bleeding time. Our hypothesis seemed to hold true. During another expedition to Greenland we found the same platelet behaviour and increased bleeding time as we expected [9].

We were rather enthousiastic about our observations in the Greenlanders. We felt that we had found the explanation of the infrequency of thrombotic diseases in the Eskimos. We wondered whether or not our observations could lead to a thrombosis prophylaxis also in other parts of the world. Several further studies of the effects of Ω-3 fatty acids with 20 or 22 carbon atoms also by other authors seem to confirm our hypothesis.

We have for a long period of time known that high levels of cholesterol in the blood induce increased risk of thrombotic diseases. Furthermore, we are aware of the fact that saturated fat in the food increases and polyunsaturated fat decreases the blood cholesterol level. But nobody had hitherto realized that there are two different sorts of polyunsaturated fatty acids with very different biological and nutritional properties, namely the fatty acids of the Ω-6 family essentially of vegetable origin, and the Ω-3 fatty acids coming from marine animals.

The Ω-3 fatty acid family seems to have special properties concerning platelet aggregation and hence as a prophylaxis against thrombotic diseases and the development of atherosclerosis.

We and other researchers carried out studies of the effects of fish oil and fish oil concentrates in animals and humans. I can only mention a few of these studies. The degree of myocardial infarction after electrical irritation of the coronary arteries in dogs was significantly less in those dogs given fish oil [10].

In swine who were made severely hypercholesterolaemic by their food the degree of atherosclerotic changes in their arteries was significantly less in those swine who got a supplementation of fish oil as compared with the control animals, even if both groups stayed in the hypercholesterolaemic state [11].

Japanese researchers examined the blood lipids in Japanese fishermen who experience a much lower incidence of thrombotic diseases than Japanese farmers who served as controls. Their observations were very similar to our Eskimo observations [12].

112

Dutch researchers, Kromhout and others, compared the mortality from ischaemic heart disease in people who eat fish with that of other people who never consumed fish during a twenty years' period. He found that as little as 30 g fish a day averagely caused a reduction of the mortality of coronary heart disease to the half [13].

Recently some studies of the frequency of restenosis after coronary angioplasty have shown some but significant reduction of this event after supplementation with fish oil [14]. Another important clinic observation published recently showed a significant decrease of the frequency of new coronary occlusion in people who have survived their first attack of this disease and who received fish oil preparations [15]. These two studies seem especially informative as the patients concerned had severe degrees of atherosclerosis, and in spite of this, fish oil still had a beneficial effect.

In Oslo, during the Second World War, a significant decrease of thrombotic and embolic diseases was observed. In order to avoid starvation, people were forced to eat fish and fish products rather exclusively because the occupation troops removed almost all animal and diary products. We could calculate from dietary reports that people during this period of time in Oslo consumed about 4-5 g EPA a day, the same amount as we found in the Greenlanders' food. After the war when the nutritional situation had returned to normal the prevalence of thrombotic diseases in Oslo increased to the pre-war level or a little above [16].

A certain bleeding tendency had been observed in the Greenland Eskimos during centuries. In an old Norse chronicle from the thirteenth century it is told that the Eskimos when killed in fight with the Norse intruders would not stop bleeding [17]. Nose bleedings, obstetric haemorrhages, haemoptyses – when pulmonary tuberculosis was still frequent – haemorrhagic ex- and enanthema in smallpox and measles and even haemolacry (erythrocytes in the tear fluid) have been observed in the Greenland Eskimos. This was hitherto unexplained. Our observation of the decreased platelet aggregability and hence increased bleeding time and tendency in the Eskimos have offered an explanation.

Since our first publications in 1978 [6, 7] several researchers have examined the properties of fish oil or concentrates both experimentally and clinically

I shall try to give a short survey of our knowledge about EPA and its virtues today : Japanese researchers have found that EPA reduces the blood viscosity [18] and increases the deformability of the red cells [19], both of importance for the rheological circumstances in the small vessels. Mild hypertension is improved by EPA [20]. EPA reduces strongly hypertriglyceridemia [21], but its reduction of hypercholesterolemia is more doubtful. It has been found that EPA ameliorates or diminishes attacks of the genuine hemicrania [22]. I myself an example of this effect. It has been shown that

EPA improves some sort of psoriasis, especially its pustulous forms [24], and atopic dermatitis. The stiffness and plains in the joints in rheumatoid arthritis are bettered by EPA [24]. Even osteoarthritis is reported to be improved by fish oil [25]. Recently it has been found that dietary cod liver oil will normalize the increased microvascular albumin leakage in diabetics with albuminuria [26]. Fish oil has been reported to have a favourable effect on the risk of thrombosis in renal allografts recipients [27]. Lupus erythematosis is improved. Preeclampsia is infrequent in Greenland Eskimos [28] and it seems that EPA can influence this disease beneficially. Several other clinical trials are being carried out in different diseases, and we will possibly learn about further beneficial effects by EPA in the future. As examples I may mention trials on Buerger's disease (preliminary results are promising), severe atherosclerosis of the lower limbs and ulcerous colitis. It seems that certains forms of cancer, for instance mammary, colon and prostate, are less frequent in populations with a high intake of fish.

One problem is still rather unsolved, namely the dose of EPA, necessary to cause clinical effect. We found that the Greenlanders consumed about 5 g EPA a day. Some preliminar non published Japanese examinations showed that a supplementation of at least 1.8-2 g EPA a day was necessary to influence beneficially Buerger's disease and severe atherosclerosis of the lower limbs. The observation of Kromhout [13] as cited before showed that even as little as 30 g fish a day caused cases of ischaemic heart disease to be halved during a 20 years' period of time. Consequently, we do not know the exact clinically necessary dose of EPA, but I would suggest that in clinical studies EPA should be given at least at 2 g a day. Furthermore, it should be remembered that docosahexaenoic acid (C 22 : 6 Ω-3), also abundant in most fish oils, in easily converted to EPA by humans. In this connexion it must be mentioned that α-linolenic acid (C 18 : 3 Ω-3), even if it belongs to the Ω-3 family, is only scarcely and slowly transformed to EPA by humans [29], while rats can do it easily.

The beneficial effect by EPA on the several conditions and diseases mentioned before and probably not explained by its effect on platelet aggregability. Since our original observations, other properties of EPA have been found. The most important are the following : the chemotaxis of monocytes and neutrophils which is important for the atherosclerotic process is hampered by EPA [30]. The anti-allergic and anti-inflammatory effects of EPA is probably explained by the production by EPA of leukotriene of the 5-family which is less active than the leucotriene of the 4-family with arachidonic as precursor [32]. The blood level of antithrombin III is enhanced by EPA causing less coagulability of the blood [32]. The decreased concentration of blood fibrinogen goes in the same direction [33]. Interleukin-1 and tumor necrosis factor are diminished by EPA causing inhibition of the coagulation factor plasminogen activator and of the proliferation of smooth muscle cells in the arterial wall during the atherosclerotic process [34].

We still do not know if supplementation of fish oil preparations or concentrates over a long period of time can have unfavourable effects in humans. However, in the many observations and experiments with EPA in humans hitherto published, no harmful effects have been observed. What we know for certain is that Greenland Eskimos in thousands of years have consumed great amounts of EPA and DHA with – as it seems – only beneficial effects.

References

1. Kromann N, Green A. Epidemiological studies in the Upernavik district, Greenland. Acta med scand 1980; 208 : 401-6.

2. Bang HO, Dyerberg J, Hjørne N. The composition of food consumed by Greenland Eskimos. Acta med Scand 1976; 200 : 69-73.

3. Bang HO, Dyeberg J. Plasma lipids and lipoproteins in Greenland westcoast Eskimos. Acta med Scand 1972; 192 : 85-94.

3. Dyeberg J, Bang HO, Hjørne N. Fatty acid composition of the plasma lipids in Greenland Eskimos. Am J Clin Nutr 1975; 28 : 958-66.

5. Keys A, Kimura N. Diets of middle-aged farmers in Japan. Am J Clin Nutr 1970; 23 : 212-23.

6. Dyeberg J, Bang HO. Dietary fat and thrombosis. Lancet 1978 : 1 : 152.

7. Dyeberg J, Bang HO, Stoffersen E *et al*. Eicosapentaenoic acid and prevention of thrombosis and atherosclerosis. Lancet 1978; 2 : 117-9.

7. Hamazaki T, Fischer S, Schweer H *et al*. The infusion of trieicopentaenoyl-glycerol into humans and the *in vivo* formation of Prostaglandin I 3 and Thromboxane A 3. Biochem Biophys Research Com 1988 : 151 1386-94.

9. Dyeberg J, Bang HO. Haemostatic function and platelet polyunsaturated fatty acids in Eskimos. Lancet 1979; 2 : 433-5.

10. Culp B, Lands WEM, Lucches BR *et al*. The effect of dietary supplementation of fish oil on experimental myocardial infarction. Prostaglandins 1980; 20 : 1021-31.

11. Weiner BH, Ockene IS, Levine PH. Inhibition of atherosclerosis by cod liver oil in hyperlipidaemic swine. N Engl J Med 1986; 315 841-6.

12. Hirai A, Hamazaki T, Terano T. Eicosapentaenoic acid and platelet function in Japanese. Lancet 1980; 2 : 1132-3.

13. Kromhout D, Bosschieter EB, de Lenzenne-Coulander C. The inverse relation between fish consumption and 20 years mortality from coronary heart disease. N Engl J Med 1985; 312 : 1205-9.

14. Dehmer GJ, Popma JJ, Berg EKVD *et al*. Reduction in the rate of early re-stenosis after coronary angioplasty by a diet supplemented with Ω-3 fatty acid. N Engl J Med 1988; 319 : 733-40.

15. Burr ML, Gilbert JF, Holliday RM *et al*. Effects of changes in fat, fish, and fibre intakes on death and myocardial reinfarction : Diet and reinfarction trial (Dart). Lancet 1989; 2 : 757-61.

16. Bang HO, Dyeberg J. Personal reflections on the incidence of ischaemic heart disease in Oslo during the Second World War. Acta med Scand 1981; 210 : 245-48.

17. Bang HO, Dyeberg J. The bleeding tendency in Greenland Eskimos. Dan Med Bull 1980; 27 : 202-5.

18. Kobayashi S, Hamazaki T, Hirai A *et al*. Epidemiological and clinical studies of the effect of eicosapentaenoic acid (EPA C 20 : 5 Ω-3) on blood viscosity. Clin Hemorheology 1985; 5 : 493-505.

19. Kamada T, Yamashita T, Baba Y *et al*. Dietary sardine oil increases erythrocyte membrane fluidity in diabetic patients. Diabetes 1986; 35 : 604-11.

20. Mortensen JZ, Schmidt EB, Nielsen AH *et al*. The effect of Ω-6 and Ω-3 polyunsaturated fatty acids on hemostasis, blood lipids and blood pressure. Thromb Haemostas (Stuttgart) 1983; 50 : 543-6.

21. Nestel PJ, Connor WE, Reardon MF *et al*. Suppression by diets rich in fish oil of very low density lipoprotein production in man. J Clin Invest 1984; 74 : 82-9.

22. McCarren TJ, Hitzemann R, Smith R *et al*. Membranes and migraine. In Olesen J, Tfelt-Hansen P, Jensen K. Proceed Second Internat Headache Congress, Copenhagen 1985 : 548.

23. Kettler AH, Baughn RE, Orengo IF *et al*. The effect of dietary fish oil supplementation on psoriasis. J Am Acad Dermatol 1988, 18 : 1267-73.

24. Kremer JM, Jubiz W, Michalek AV *et al*. Fish oil fatty acid supplementation in active rheumatoid arthritis. Ann Intern Med 1987; 106 : 497-503.

25. Stammers T, Sibbald B, Freding P. Fish oil and osteoarthritis. Lancet 1989; 2 : 503.

26. Jensen T, Stender S, Goldstein K *et al*. Partial normalization by dietary cod-liver oil of increased microvascular albumin leakage in patients with insulin-dependent diabetes and albuminuria. N Engl J Med 1989; 321 : 1572-7.

27. Urakaze M, Hamazaki T, Kashiwabara H *et al*. Favourable effects of fish oil concentrate on risk factors for thrombosis in renal allograft recipients. Nephron 1989; 53 : 102-9.

28. Dyeberg J, Bang HO. Pre-eclampsia and prostaglandins. Lancet 1985; 1 : 1267.

29. Dyeberg J, Bang HO, Aagaard O. α-linolenic acid and eicosapentaenoic acid, Lancet 1980; 1 : 199.

30. Schmidt EB, Pedersen PO, Ekelund S *et al*. Cod liver oil inhibits neutrophil and monocyte chemotaxis in healthy males. Atherosclerosis 1989; 77 : 53-7.

31. Lee TH, Austen KF. Arachidonic acid metabolism by the 5-lipoxygenase pathway, and the effects of alternative dietary fatty acid. Adv Immunology 1986; 39 : 145-75.

32. Stoffersen E, Jørgensen KA, Dyeberg J. Antithrombin III and dietary intake of polyunsaturated fatty acids. Scand J Clin Lab Invest 1982; 42 : 83-6.

33. Høstmark AT, Bjerkedal T, Kierulf P *et al*. Fish oil and plasma fibrinogen. Brit Med J 1988; 297 : 180-1.

34. Endres S, Ghorbani R, Kelley VE *et al*. The effect of dietary supplementation with Ω-3 polyunsaturated fatty acids on the synthesis of Interleukin-1 and tumor necrosis factor by mononuclear cells. N Engl J Med 1989; 320 : 268-71.

Fish oil and blood-vessel wall interactions. Eds P.M. Vanhoutte, Ph. Douste-Blazy.
John Libbey Eurotext, Paris © 1991, pp. 117-127.

12

Lipoprotein particles : clinical significance

J.C. Fruchart

*Serlia and U. INSERM 325, Pasteur Institute,
1, Rue du Président Calmette, Lille.*

A certain number of techniques for the separation of lipoproteins according to their physico-chemical properties, have been suggested. It has, however, recently been shown that lipoproteins defined in terms of physico-chemical properties (VLDL, IDL, LDL and HDL) are in fact, from a chemical and metabolical viewpoint, homogenious entities. According to Alaupovic's concept, plasma lipoproteins consist of a mixture of particles each of which is characterised by a particular protein composition.

With the use of specific dosage techniques (immuno-enzymology with dual anti-body determination and differential electro-immunodiffusion) we have been able to show that determining particle characteristics is essential to the clarification of the diagnostic value of AI and B apolipoprotein dosage. The metabolism of lipoprotein particles containing apo A-I or apo B seems to be affected primarily by their corresponding protein composition. Certain sub-categories of lipoprotein particles containing apo B, such as LpB, a particle containing only apo B, LpB : E containing apo B and E, LpB : C-III, and Lp(a) : B containing apo (a) and B, have been identified as significant atherogenous risk factors.

We have also recently shown that the protective effect attributed to HDLs was due to the LpA-Is particles containing apo A-I but not apo A-II, while LpA-1 : A-II containing apo A-I and A-II had little or no effect. Dyslipoproteinaemias are characterised by the different characteristics of the particles

117

containing apo B. Distribution anomalies of particles containing apo A-I are connected, in the case of young children, to a family history of coronary disease and could explain differences in coronary mortality in different populations. In addition hypolipemia drugs seem to effect particles containing apo B and containing apo A-I in a particular way.

The majority of metabolical, clinical and epidemiological studies carried out in the last 30 years, are based on a physico-chemical system of lipoprotein classification.

Electrophoresis, floatation ultracentrifugation and more recently selective precipitation techniques have made possible a somewhat arbitrary separation of often very closely related fractions. The classification of dyslipoproteinaemias was for a long time based on this approach, but recent work, in particular that undertaken in our laboratory, has cast a shadow on its validity, by illustrating the metabolical heterogeneity of lipoproteins defined using standard classification techniques [1]. In fact the particles isolated by standard techniques are not homogeneous from a molecular viewpoint and correspond to a mixture of distinct lipoprotein particles each of whose clinical significance is different [2]. Along the lines of P. Alaupovic we recently suggested a lipoprotein classification technique based on their protein composition. The development of reliable and sufficiently simple immunological techniques has allowed us to introduce lipoprotein particle dosage into the repertory of routine examinations employed in clinical biochemistry. The results obtained and outlined in this paper should be an encouragement to the biologist and the clinician to use lipoprotein particle analysis both as a criterion in diagnosis and as a highly sensitive control technique for the efficiency of normo-lipoprotein therapies.

Suggested technique for a system of lipoprotein classification based on apoliprotein composition

The specific chemical and immunological characteristics of apolipoproteins make them ideal indicators for a molecular definition of lipoproteins. Apolipoproteins could be said to represent the intelligent faculties of lipoproteins in so far as they make possible their receptor interaction, and regulate the activity of the enzymes involved in their metabolism *(Table 1)*.

By obtaining the specific antibodies of each apolipoprotein it was possible to establish the immunological characteristics of lipoproteins which can be

Table I. Properties and functions of apolipoproteins in HDL.

Apolipoproteins								
Serum concentrations (mg/ml)								
Molecular weight (10) dattoms								
Number of amino-acids								
Synthesis sites	Liver Intestine	Liver Intestine	Liver Intestine	Liver	Liver Intestine	Liver	Gonads, kidneys placenta, liver, intestine	Liver, intestine, scanenger cells, muscles
Chromosome gene localisation								
Functions	LcAT activator Ligand for «NDL» receptor Activator for reverse cholesterol transport	Ligand for «HDL» receptor Inhibitor of % reverse cholesterol transport	LCAt activator Ligand for «NDL» receptor Activator for reverse cholesterol transport	LCAT activator (?)	LPL activator	LPL inhibitor	Possible role in cholesterol ester metabolism	Ligand for apo E and B/E receptors

considered as a mixture of distinct lipoprotein particles each one possessing a specific protein composition *(Figure 1)* :

- single particles, made up of a combination of lipids and an apoprotein (e.g. LpB which contains exclusively apolipoprotein B);

- complex particles, a combination of lipids plus two or several apolipoproteins (e.g. LpB : C-III : E, which contains, in the same particle, apolipoproteins B, C-III, E).

Each family of particles in fact represents a poly-dispersal system. Thus LpB can be found in VLDL, IDL or LDL, according to the lipid protein ratio within the particle [4].

A lipo-particle defined in terms of its apolipoprotein content, possesses specific functions and could represent the basic unit of lipid metabolism. Thus, for example, the definition of apolipoprotein B varies according to the lipo-particles with carries it. Lipo-particles containing apolipoprotein B combined with apolipoprotein E are very readily recognized by the LDL-receptor, while those containing a combination of apolipoproteins B and C-III, or B and (a) are less easily recognisable *(Figure 2)*.

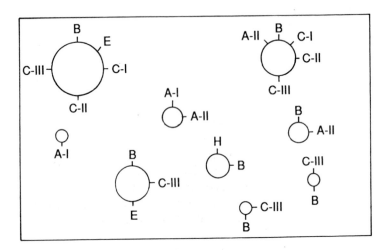

Figure 1. Lipoprotein particle diagram. Classification by apolipoprotein composition. (Based on P. Alaupovic).

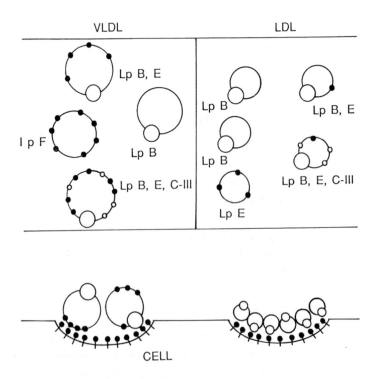

Figure 2. Cell/lipo-particle interaction diagram.

We have also been able to show recently that particles LP A-I and LP A-I : A-II are metabolically distinct. Particles LP A-I alone are responsible for the cholesterol out-flow in the case of reverse cholesterol transport from peripheral tissues to the liver [7].

The very considerable recent progress in lipoprotein biology now makes it possible to consider a classification technique based on the functionally significant epitopes which are accessible on the surface of a given lipo-particle. An apolipoprotein such as apolipoprotein B can be compared to an «iceberg» floating on a sea of oil. One part is visible and accessible on the surface of the molecule while another part is hidden under the lipids. The epitopes present on the surface are different according to the lipid make-up and whether or not one or several combined apolipoproteins are present within the same particle. On the other hand a given epitope can be modified by genetic mutation, as in the case, for example, of that corresponding to amino-acid 3500 of apo B, and which results in the failure of the LDL receptor to recognize the lipo-particle [8]. The recent introduction of monoclone antibodies allows us to differenciate and even, in certain cases, to quantify, lipo-particles in terms of accessible epitopes [9].

Lipo-particle quantification

There are two methodologies currently in use in routine clinical biochemistry for the dosage of lipo-particles.

Immuno-enzymology with dual anti-body determination, which consists in «sandwiching» the particle to be dosed between one insolubilized anti-body on a solid phase and a second anti-body with an enzyme indicator. This technique allows us to quantify particles containing A-II and A-I [10] (a) and B [11], E and B, C-III and B [12] *(Figure 3)*.

The use of a suitably chosen anti-B monoclonal anti-body as the first anti-body and a polyclonal anti-body or a mixture of anti-B monoclonal antibodies in order to reveal the particles containing apo B in terms of epitope accessibility *(Figure 3)*. A change in an amino-acid within an epitope or a modification of the lipid and/or protein environment can thus decrease the affinity between the lipo-particle and the anti-body [9, 13].

The differential electro-immunodiffusion is another favoured technique for lipo-particle dosage. If the serum to be dosed contains two groups of lipo-particles containing the same apolipoprotein Y and one of these groups processes concomitantly another apolipoprotein Z, then, in order to bring

121

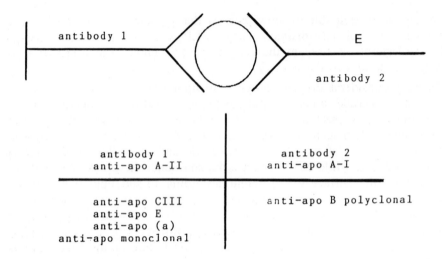

Figure 3. Particle determination using immuno-enzymology with dual antibody determination.

about a differential dosage, two different anti-bodies are mixed in a gel with one being preponderant (in this case with a preponderance of anti-Z).

During migration the lipo-particles containing Y and Z are blocked in the gel creating an initial peak, while those which contain only Y continue to migrate and subsequently create a second precipitation peak whose height (or surface area) is proportional to the concentration in the serum of the Y-charged (but not the Z-charged) particles.

For example, the introduction into a gel of anti apo A-I antibodies and of a considerable preponderance of anti-apo A-II antibodies allows us to dose the lipo-particles containing A-I and not A-II (LP A-I) [14]. In the same way, the introduction into a gel of anti-apo E (or anti-apo C-III) anti-bodies and a considerable preponderance of anti-apo AI, permits the dosage of lipo-particles containing E (or C-III) but not containing A-1 (LP B-E, LPB-C-III).

Clinical significance of the dosage of lipo-particles containing apolipoproteina-I

HDL contain two main types of lipoprotein particles which we have recently characterised [15]:
- lipo-particles containing both apolipoproteins A-I and A-II (LP A-I : A-II) mainly found in HDL3 and synthesised by the liver;

- lipo-particles containing apolipoprotein A-I but not A-11 (LP A-I) mainly found in HDL2 and synthesised by the intestin and the liver; it is interesting to note that apoliprotein A-IV, lecithin-cholesterol-acyl-transferase and cholesterol transfer protein, which all play a part in the reverse transfer of cholesterol are most frequently found in LP A-I [16].

While these two particle types are metabolically distinct, the overall assessment of apo A-I allows us to analyse them only as a whole; a decrease of apo A-I for example could reflect a decrease of LP A-I and/or LP A-I : A-II. Thanks to the techniques described above, we have recently been able to asseses the respective LP A-I and LP A-I : A-II serum concentrations in specific psychopathological conditions. We showed, first of all, that the increase in apo A-I serum concentration in human female (as opposed to male) subjects is linked to LP A-I and not to LP A-I : A-II [14]. A recent study on angiography subjects showed that subjects withy angiographic atherosclerosis have LP A-I serum concentrations significantly lower than those of control subjects while those with LP A-I : A-II are unchanged [17].

A study undertaken jointly with the Moscow Institute of Cardiology shows clearly that LP A-I is the clearest indicator for the differenciation of adolescents in terms of cardiovascular family history [18].

All these results underline the anti-atherogenous role of LP A-I and are further corroborated by a study jointly undertaken with Professor Davignon and his collaborators (Clinical Research Institute of Montreal) among average age and octogenerian subjects have significantly increased LP A-I serum concentrations, while their apo A-I serum concentrations are lower [19] *(Table II)*.

Table II. LP A-1 in octogenarians.

	Normolipemia n = 68		Octogenarians n = 168	
	Women	Men	Women	Men
Age (in years)	37.5 ± 6.7	38.2 ± 6.9	83.9 ± 3.3	84.8 ± 4.5
LP A-I (mg/dl)	56.8 ± 11.3*	51.0 ± 9.8*	67.2 ± 14.9*	59.4 ± 7.1*

*p < 0.001.

These studies taken together underline the value of examining different HDL particles. This value is further increased by the fact that we have recently been able to show that LP A-I, LP A-I : A-II and cholesterol HDL concentrations could vary inversely under the effect of medication of nutrition. It was thus that, while assessing these parameters in subjects consuming varying amounts of a alcohol, we observed that an increase in HDL cholesterol

% variation

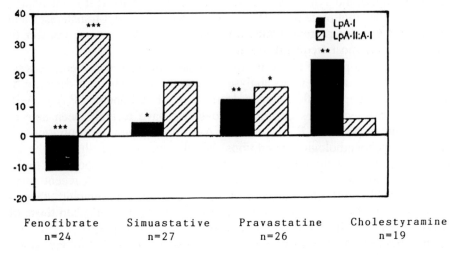

*p < 0.05;   **P < 0.01; ***p < 0.001 ;   Wilcoxon test administrated / placebo

Figure 4. Medication effects on lipoprotein particles containing apolipoprotein A-I.

was connected to that of LP A-I : A-II, concealing a decrease in LP A-I, previously defined as being the anti-atherogenous fraction of HDL [20]. The same assessment applied to subjects undergoing hypolipemia therapy shows again a dissociation between fibrates, which considerably increase LP A-I A-II, but which decrease LP A-I, and resins or HMGCoA reductase inhibitors which increase both fractions [21] *(Figure 4)*.

Dosage of lipoprotein particles therefore seems to reflect more accurately the complexity of high density lipoprotein metabolism, which can now be more comprehensively understood, since the discovery and purification of HDL receptors [22].

Clinical significance of the dosage of lipo-particles containing apolipoprotein B

Lipo-particles containing apolipoprotein B are heterogeneous and their independent dosage has become indispensable for the diagnosis and follow-up of dyslipoproteinemia.

Lipo-particles separated according to their apolipoprotein composition

The most numerous lipo-particles are those containing apolipoprotein B exclusively of any other apolipoprotein (LpB). It is these whose concentration increases in the plasma of subjects affected by familial hypercholesterolemia [23]. They are particularly sensitive to the action of HMG CoA reductase inhibitors [23].

Lipo-particles containing apolipoprotein B and apolipoprotein C-III form part of the residual particles created during VLDL and chylomicron catabolism. They build up in renal deficiency hemodialysis subjects [24] in type II diabetes. We have recently been able to confirm their atherogenicity in an (unpublished) retrospective epidemiological study carried out on angiography subjects. They are more sensitive to fibrates than to HMG CoA reductase inhibitors [25, 26].

Lipo-particles containing apolipoprotein B and apolipoprotein E similarly form part of the residual particles resulting from the catabolism of lipoproteins rich in triglycerides.

They have a particular tendency to build up in type III dyslipoproteinemia, where there is both hypersynthesis and an apo E recognition anomaly on the part of its genetic receptor.

Practically all B lipo-particles in this case are combined with E and the dosage of B : E particles is pathognomonic of this condition [27].

B : E particles are highly atherogenous and are found in increased density in patients with coronary atherosclerosis, even if total plasma apo B concentration is normal. They are more sensitive to fibrates than to HMG CoA reductase inhibitors [25, 27].

Lipo-particles containing apolipoprotein B and apolipoprotein (a) or LP (a) are genetically controlled. They are present in atheromous platelets and a serum concentration of over 30 mg/l is an independent risk factor for atherosclerosis and thrombosis which should be looked for.

A remarkable homology between apolipoprotein (a) and plasminogen has recently been discovered [28]. Competition between Lp (a) and plasminogen for plasminogen receptors [29, 30] could explain the thrombogenous and atherogenous powers of Lp (a).

References

1. Puchois P, Alaupovic P, Fruchart JC. Mise au point sur les classifications des lipoprotéines plasmatiques. Ann Biol Clin 1985; 43 : 831-840.

2. Fruchart JC, Koffigan M, Fievet C *et al*. Molecular analysis of lipoproteins. Clinical applications. Lipoproteins and Atherosclerosis, Plenum Press, Eds Malmendier CL and Alaupovic P, 1987; pp 225-231.

3. Fruchart JC. Polyclonal, oligoclonal and monoclonal antibody mapping of the lipoprotein particles. *In : Proceedings of the 7th international atherosclerosis symposium,* Elsevier Science Publishers, Atherosclerosis VII, Eds. Fidge and Nestel, 1986; pp. 287-290.

4. Alaupovic P, Tavella M, Fesmire J. Separation and identification of apo B containing lipoprotein particles in normolipemic subjects and patients with hyperlipoproteinemias. *In : Lipoproteins and atherosclerosis,* Plenum Press, Eds CL Malmendier and P Alaupovic, 1987; pp 7-14.

5. Agnani G, Clavey V, Candelier L *et al*. Influence de la composition en apolipoprotéines des lipoprotéines sur leur affinité pour le récepteur B/E des cellules HeLa. *In : Biologie Prospective, comptes rendus du 7e Colloque de Pont-à-Mousson,* John Libbey Eurotext, Eds. MM Galteau, Siest G, Henny J, 1989; pp 161-164.

6. Gries A, Fievet C, Marcovina S *et al*. Interaction of LDL, Lp (a) and reduced Lp (a) with monoclonal antibodies against apo B J Lipid Res *et al*. 1988; 29 : 1-8.

7. Barbaras R, Puchois P, Fruchart JC *et al*. Cholesterol efflux from cultured adipose cells is mediated by LpA-I particles but not by LpA-1 : A-II particles. Biochem Biophys Res Commun 1987; 142(1) : 63-69.

8. Innerarity TL, Weisgraber KH, Arnold KS *et al*. Familial defective apolipoprotein B-100 : low density lipoproteins with abnormal receptor binding. Proc Natl Acad Sci USA 1987; 84; 6919-6923.

9. Luyeye I, Fievet C, Dupont JC *et al*. Human apolipoprotein B. Evidence for its immunochemical heterogeneity using monoclonal antibodies and an immunoenzymometric assay. Clin Biochem 1988; 21 : 255-261.

10. Koren E, Puchois P, Alaupovic P *et al*. Quantitative determination of two different types of apolipoproteins particles in human plasma by an enzyme linked differential antibody immunoabsorbent assay. Clin Chem 1987; 33 : 38-43.

11. Vu-Dac N, Mezdour H, Parra HJ *et al*. A selective bisite immunoenzymometric procedure for human Lp (a) lipoprotein quantification using monoclonal antibodies against apo (a) and apo BJ Lipid Res 1989; 30 : 1437-1443.

12. Fruchart JC, Kandoussi A, Parsy D *et al*. Measurement of lipoprotein particles defined by their apolipoprotein composition using immunoabsorbent assay. Annual meeting on clinical chemistry, Mannheim, September 25-28, 1985, (abstr), J Clin Chem Clin Biochem, 1985; 23 : 619.

13. Duriez P, Butler R, Tikkanen MJ *et al*. A monoclonal antibody (BIP 45) detects Ag (c,g) polymorphism of human apolipoprotein B. J Immunol Meth 1987; 102 : 205-212.

14. Parra HJ, Mezdour H, Ghalim N *et al*. Differential electroimmunoassay on ready-to-use plates for human LpA-I lipoprotein particles. Clin Chem 1989, accepté pour publication.

15. Barkia A, Puchois P, Ghalim N *et al.* Differential role apolipoprotein A-1 containing particles in cholesterol efflux from adipose cells. Arteriosclerosis, 1989, soumis à publication.

16. Puchois P, Steinmetz A, Ghalim N *et al.* Characterization of apolipoproteins containing apo A-I but not apo A-II from human interstitial fluid. Circulation, 1988; 78 : (4), 168 (abstract 0665).

17. Puchois P, Kandoussi A, Fievet P *et al.* Apolipoprotein A-I containing lipoproteins in coronary artery disease Arteriosclerosis, 1987; 68 : 35-40.

18. Metelskaya V, Aingorn H, Bard JM *et al.* Apolipoprotein A-I containing lipoproteins in children with positive family history of coronary heart disease, 1989, soumis à publication.

19. Luc G, Bard JM, Lussier-Cacan S *et al.* High density lipoprotein particles in octogenarians. Metabolism, 1989, soumis à publication.

20. Puchois P, Ghalim N, Demarquilly C *et al.* Effect of alcohol consumption on lipoprotein particles which contain apo A-I and apo A-II (LpA-I : A-II) and apo A-I but not apo A-II (LpA-I). Circulation, 1986; 74; (4), 383 (abstract 1528).

21. Fruchart JC, Bard JM, Puchois P *et al.* Clinical significance of apo A-I containing lipoprotein particles. *In : Proceedings of the 8th international symposium on atherosclerosis,* Rome, october 9-13, 1988, Experta Medica, Atherosclerosis VIII, Eds G Crepaldi, AM Gotto, E Manzato, G Baggio, 1989, pp 395-398.

22. Barbaras R, Puchois P, Fruchart JC *et al.* Purification of the apolipoprotein. A receptor from mouse adipose cells. J Biol Clin 1989, soumis à publication.

23. Alaupovic P, Tavella M, Corder CN *et al.* Selective effect of hypolipidemic drugs on discrete apo B containing lipoprotein particles. International atherosclerosis congress, Vienna, april 20-21, 1989.

24. Parsy D, Dracon M, Cachera C *et al.* Lipoprotein abnormalities in chronic hemodialysis patients. Nephrol Dialys Trans 1988; 3 : 51-56.

25. Fruchart JC, Bard JM, Fievet C *et al.* Effect of fenofibrate on apolipoprotein B containing lipoprotein particles. *In : Recent aspects of diagnosis and treatment of lipoprotein disorders : impact on prevention of atherosclerosis diseases.* Ed AR Liss, 1988; pp 305-310.

26. Bard JM, Luc G, Douste-Blazy P *et al.* Effect of simvastatin on lipids apolipoproteins and lipoprotein particles in primary hypercholesterolemia. *In : Atherosclerosis reviews,* Eds Stockes J III and Mancini M, Raven Press, 1988; pp 153.160.

27. Fruchart JC, Davignon J, Bard JM *et al.* Effect of fenofibrate treatment on type III hyperlipoproteinemia, Amer J Med, 1987, 83; (5B), 71-74.

28. McLean JW, Tomlinson JE, Kuang WJ *et al.* cDNA sequence of human apolipoprotein (a) in homologous to plasminogen. Nature 1987; 330 : 132-137.

29. Miles LA, Fless GM, Levin EG *et al.* A potential basis for the thrombotic risk associated with lipoprotein (a). Nature 1989; 339; 301-303.

30. Hajjar KA, Gravish D, Breslow JL *et al.* Lipoprotein (a) modulation of endothelial cell surface fibrinolysis ans its potential role in atheroclerosis. Nature 1989; 339 : 303-305.

Fish oil and blood-vessel wall interactions. Eds P.M. Vanhoutte, Ph. Douste-Blazy.
John Libbey Eurotext, Paris © 1991, pp. 129-131.

13

Ω-3 fatty acid and diabetes mellitus

F. Berthezene

Department of Endocrinology and Nutritional Disease
Lipid Metabolism Laboratory
INSERM U197, Antiquaille Hospital, Lyon, France.

Abstract

Bearing in mind the potentially advantageous effects of Ω-3 fatty acid in sugar diabetes these results should not lead to their rejection but should rather prompt further studies along three main lines :
1. the definition of the minimal efficient posology and the types of patients who are more susceptible to respond to this treatment without harmful secondary effects;
2. the transformation mechanisms, in particular on the LDL metabolism and on the cholesterol return route;
3. it is finally indispensable that random prospective studies be undertaken to improve our understanding of the effect of Ω-3 fatty acids on cardiovascular morbidity and mortality in diabetic patients.

Diabetes mellitus is common. For example, the number of diabetic patients in France is estimated at 1 000 000 to 1 500 000. Mainly as a result of the increased incidence and seriousness of arterial atheroma (particularly of coronary arteries) the life expectancy of these subjects is reduced [1]. The development of coronary disease in diabetic patients is due to the influence of numerous factors; these include : glucosylation of circulating or structural proteins, hypertriglyceridemia (the most reliable prediction factor for the risk of atheroma) [2], and accentuated platelet aggregation. The consumption of Ω-3 fatty acids by the diabetic patient is therefore potentially very advantageous given the decreasing effect of these fatty acids on circulating triglycerides and on platelet aggregation, and their ability to improve the glycemia balance (Greenland Eskimos rarely suffer from diabetes mellitus in spite of the frequency of obesity). It would also appear that eicosanoidal acids play a part *in the cholesterol outflow from cells to the HDL [3]*. Moreover this outflow is considerably impaired by non insulin dependent diabetes mellitus. The effect of Ω-3 fatty acids on platelet activity in diabetic subjects is well known. We have demonstrated that doses as low as 50 mg per day diminish collagen induced platelet aggregation in these patients [4]. The fatty acids have a direct effect on the myocardium since, when administered to the diabetic rat, they prevent the development of cardiomyopathy [5]. They also act directly on the arterial walls, diabetic subjects who regularly consume fish having less significant peripheral arterial resistance than those who do not [6]. It has also been demonstrated that the administration of fish liver oil improves both blood pressure reading and microvascular albumin leakage in insulin dependent diabetic patients.

Given these results, the use of Ω-3 fatty acids in diabetes mellitus appeared both advantageous and harmless. However several secondary effects connected particularly with the glycemia balance and LDL cholesterol concentration quickly became apparent and several recent publications have emphasised the possible risk involved in using these fatty acids for diabetic patients [8-9].

In fact, even if studies have shown a net reduction of triglyceride concentration in the diabetic after Ω-3 fatty acid diet supplementation, there has often, but not always, been a degradation of the glycemia balance [11-14]. This is particularly apparent in the case of non-insulin dependent diabetics, and even more so when compounded by obesity; the quantity of Ω-3 fatty acids ingested would appear to be a crucial point, increased glycemia generally becoming apparent with posologies of over 7 g per day. The mechanism of this aggravation is unknown; the fatty acids could act directly on the beta cell of the Langerhans islands and/or cause deterioration through increased energy supply. At the same time several authors have noticed an increase in LDL cholesterol and in apoprotein B, whose mechanism is again unknown.

References

1. Ekoe JM. Aspect of the world-wide of diabetes mellitus and its long-term complications. *In : Diabetes mellitus*, Ed Elsevier, Amsterdam, New York, Oxford, 1988.
2. Fontbonne A, Eschwege E, Cambien F *et al.* Hypertriglyceridaemia as a risk factor of coronary heart disease mortality in subjects with imparied glucose tolerance or diabetes. Diabetologia 1989; 32 : 300-304.

3. Pomerantz KB, Hajjar DP. Eicosanoids in regulation of arterial smooth muscle cell phenotype, proliferative capacity, and cholesterol metabolism. Arteriosclerosis 1989; 9 : 413-429.

4. Velardo B, Lagarde M, Guichardant M *et al.* Decrease of platelet activity after intake of small amounts of eicosapentaenoic acid in diabetics. Thromb Haemostas 1982; 48 : 344.

5. Black SC, Katz S, McNeill JH. Cardiac performance and plasma lipids of Ω-3 fatty acid-treated streptozocin-induced diabetic rats. Diabetes 1989, 38 : 969-974.

6. Wahlqvist ML, Lo CS, Myers KA. Fish intake and arterial wall characteristics in healthy people and diabetic patients. The Lancet 1989; 944-946.

7. Jensen T, Stender S, Goldstein K *et al.* Partial normalization by dietary cod-liver oil of increased microvascular albumin leakage in patients with insulin-dependent diabetes and albuminuria. New Engl J Med 1989; 321 : 1572-1577.

8. Sorisky A, Robbins DC. Fish oil and diabetes. The next effect. Diabetes Care 1989; 12 : 302-304.

9. Axelrod L. Perspectives in diabetes. Ω-3 fatty acids in diabetes mellitus. Gift from the sea ? Diabetes 1989; 38 : 539-543.

10. Popp-Snijders C, Schouten JA, Heine RJ *et al.* Dietary supplementation of Ω-3 polyunsaturated fatty acid improves insulin sensitivity in non-insulin-dependent diabetes. Diabetes Res 1987; 4 : 141-147.

11. Friday KE, Childs MT, Tsunehara CH *et al.* Elevated plasma glucose and lowered triglyceride levels from Ω-3 fatty acid supplementation in type II diabetes. Diabetes Care 1989; 12 : 276-281.

12. Schectman G, Kaul S, Kissebah AH. Effect of fish oil concentrate on lipoprotein composition in NIDDM. Diabetes 1988; 37 : 1567-573.

13. Glauber H, Wallace P, Griver K *et al.* Adverse metabolism effect of Ω-3 fatty acid in non-insulin-dependent diabetes mellitus. Ann Intern Med 1988; 108 : 663-668.

14. Borkman M, Chisholm DJ, Furler SM *et al.* Effects of fish oil supplementation on glucose and lipid metabolism in NIDDM. Diabetes 1989; 38 : 1314-1319.

Fish oil and blood-vessel wall interactions. Eds P.M. Vanhoutte, Ph. Douste-Blazy.
John Libbey Eurotext, Paris © 1991, pp. 133-139.

14

Ω-3 fatty acids
and risk of atherosclerosis

R. Lorenz

Medizinische Klinik Innenstadt der Universität, Munich, Germany.

A causal or at least accelerating role of dietary fat in the development of atherosclerosis has long and almost generally been accepted by laymen as well as health professionals. An apparent violation of this popular view triggered the scientific interest in Ω-3 fatty acids : native Greenland Eskimos have a very low risk of atherosclerotic vascular disease although their diet is high in total fat, low in linoleic type polyunsaturated fatty acids and relatively high in cholesterol. In a series of pioneering studies Bang and Dyeberg established that Eskimos had a favorable pattern of plasma lipids, a bleeding tendency due to low platelet reactivity, a high intake of otherwise scarce long chain Ω-3 fatty acids from their marine diet, unusually high levels of these Ω-3 fatty acids and low levels of arachidonic acid in their cell membrane phospholipids. The Ω-3 fatty acid eicosapentaenoic acid (EPA) unlike arachidonic acid (AA) did not trigger platelet aggregation. Fast growing research on Ω-3 fatty acids during the last decade has meanwhile revealed several lines of evidence that relate Ω-3 fatty acids to a low risk of atherosclerotic vascular disease.

Epidemiologic studies

Despite earlier occasional reports [1], broad attention was drawn to the association of a largely marine based diet with a low incidence of atherosclerotic vascular complications only by Bang and Dyeberg [2]. Their observation was confirmed by a systematic epidemiologic survey in another district of Greenland [3]. Westernized Eskimos living in Denmark appeared to have also a western pattern of morbidity, thus implicating a peristatic rather than a genetic factor. However, comparison of an arctic hunter population with western industrial societies has to take into account many potential important differences in life style. A less exotic example is provided by Japan, where also fish intake is traditionally high and atherothrombotic cardiovascular disease is low, but increased with the adoption of western nutritional habits [4].

These transcultural comparisons were later supplemented with cross-sectionnal studies comparing patients with cardiovascular disorders to healthy subjects selected from the same population. In one such case control study the risk of new onset angina was estimated to increase 20 % for a 0.1 % decrease in EPA content of platelet membranes. The relation of EPA content to a first myocardial infarction was less clear [5].

Longitudinal evidence for a protective effect of Ω-3 fatty acid came from historical observations and the reevaluation of several prospective studies on risk factors. The forced change in dietary intake to more fish and less total fat in Oslo during Second World War was paralleled by a decline in the incidence of ischemic heart disease [6]. An inverse dose response relation was also observed between fish consumption and death from coronary heart disease during 20 years of follow-up in the Zutphen part of the Seven Countries Study [7]. Coronary mortality was reduced for more than 50 % in subjects eating 30 g fish per day. A similar result was observed by relating a 1967 dietary survey of the Swedish twin registry to the 1969 through 1982 death rates [8]. Even a lower total mortality with increasing fish consumption was reported in the reevaluation of the Western Electric study [9]. No relation of coronary death rates to fish consumption was observed in two further dietary surveys from Norway and Hawaii [10, 11]. Higher fish intake was associated with better preserved arterial compliance indicative or less sclerotic changes [12].

Effects of Ω-3 fatty acids on conventional cardiovascular risk indicators

Dyeberg first demonstrated the favourable lipid pattern in native Eskimos with low triglyceride, low density lipoprotein and very low density lipoprotein concentrations [13], whereas westernized Eskimos has lipid patterns comparable to Danes. A recent combined overview of numerous studies in healthy and hyperlipidemic subjects concluded that a major triglyceride lowering action due to reduced hepatic triglyceride synthesis and a minor increase in high density lipoprotein cholesterol could generally be demonstrated, whereas a lowering effect on the low density lipoprotein cholesterol might be due to an inadvertant reduction of saturated fat intake [14].

We could demonstrate that the blood pressure and the response to pressor hormones are significantly reduced by dietary Ω-3 fatty acids [15]. This was observed also in essential hypertensives [16] and later confirmed even in comparison to a control group on increased Ω-6 linoleic acid intake [17]. In hyperlipidemic non-insulin dependent diabetics Ω-3 fatty acid supplementation had similar effects as in non-diabetics [18], but is had adverse effects on plasma lipid pattern in normolipidemic diabetics and deteriorated glucose tolerance [19]. In type I diabetics lipids were improved [20].

Other potential protective actions of Ω-3 fatty acids

Nemerous *in vitro,* animal and human studies have addressed the effects of dietary Ω-3 fatty acids on cellular functions and biochemical pathway of potential pathogenetic or protective significance for atherogenesis [21] : EPA substitutes for AA at binding sites in plasma membrane phospholipids, is released concomitant with AA, competes for cyclooxygenase and lipoxygenase and is converted to 3 series prostaglandins and 5 series leukotrienes with a favorable spectrum of biologic actions. EPA derived TXA3 does not aggregate platelets, LTB5 is less chemotactic than LTB4, whereas PG13 formed in the vessel wall is fully active [22, 23]. *In vivo,* platelet reactivity is reduced [24], PGI3 is formed without reduction in PG12, whereas little TXA3 is formed and TXA2 is reduced after Ω-3 supplementation [25]. Both Ω-3 fatty acids, EPA and docosahexaenoic acid have antiplatelet effects [26] and very low doses may do so [27].

A second major mechanism of endothelial thromboresistance, EDRF is enhanced [28] and peptide mediators of monocyte adhesion on endothelium, like Interleukin 1 and tumor necrosis factor, are reduced [29].

The mediator of intimal smooth muscle cell immigration and proliferation, platelet derived growth factor, is reduced also [30].

The fibrinolytic capacity is increased and inhibitors of plasminogen activator and antiplasmin are reduced [31, 32]. However, also increased inhibitor has been reported [33]. Other effects of Ω-3 fatty acids include reduction of platelet activating factor, reduced plasma viscosity, increased cell deformability, reduced production of oxygen free radicals and lipid hydroperoxides [34].

Effects in animal models of atherosclerosis

Ω-3 supplementation prevented intimal hyperplasia in autologous arterialised venous implants in the dog and did so even better than antiplatelet drugs [35]. In a hypercholesterolemic swine model Ω-3 were protective against intimal hyperplasia even in the absence of a reduction in cholesterol levels [36]. A similar effect was also observed in non-human primates [37]. In a rabbit model with extreme hypercholesterolemia, however, an increase of early lesions of arteriosclerosis was observed after dietary Ω-3 addition [38].

Interventional studies with Ω-3 fatty acids in human atherosclerosis

In patients with peripheral vascular disease dietary Ω-3 fatty acids reduced elevated *in vivo* thromboxane A2 and prostacyclin formation, supposed to indicate continued pathologic platelet vessel wall interaction [39]. In an open long-term trial, a reduced nitrate demand in stable angina was reported, a finding not confirmed in a short controlled trial [40, 41]. A significantly reduced recurrence of coronary stenosis after angioplasty was reported in 3 of 5 randomised trials with Ω-3 fatty acids [42-46]. In all trials pretreatment with Ω-3 fatty acids before angioplasty may have been to short for an optimal effect. The most compelling evidence for a risk reduction by intake of Ω-3 fatty acids comes from a recent trial testing two conventional dietary recommendations, low total fat intake with P/S ratio and high fibre intake, against a high fish intake in patients recovering from myocardial infarction [47]. Only fish intake was associated with a significant reduction in cardiovascular and all cause and coronary mortality of about 30 %. This puts Ω-3 fatty acid intake among the rare pharmacological interventions shown to reduce total mortality in this setting.

Conclusion

Transcultural, cross-sectional and reevaluated longitudinal studies have in most cases confirmed the association of Ω-3 fatty acid intake with a lowered incidence of atherothrombotic disease, a hypothesis originally derived from the unique experiment of nature in native living Eskimos. Ω-3 fatty acids generally attenuate the most relevant classical risk factors, may be with the exception of type II diabetes. Ω-3 fatty acids attenuate many cellular functions and biochemical mediators implicated in atherogenesis and enhance protective mechanisms of the vessel wall. In various animal models of atherosclerosis impressive effects were seen. In man accelerated atherosclerosis resulting in restenosis after angioplasty was significantly reduced in 3 of 5 trials, despite a probably suboptimal protocol for Ω-3 fatty acid use. Ω-3 fatty acids significantly and considerably reduced total mortality after infarction, whereas two current popular dietary interventions were without effect. Benefit from a moderate increase of Ω-3 fatty acids is therefore supported by both epidemiologic observations, a plausible biologic concept and most controlled clinical trials.

References

1. Ehrström MC. Medical studies in North Greenland 1948-1949. Acta Med Scand 1951; 140 : 416-22.
2. Bang HO, Dyeberg J. Plasma lipids and lipoproteins in Greenland west coast Eskimos. Acta Med Scand 1972; 192 : 85-94.
3. Kroman N, Green A. Epidemiologic studies in the Upernavic District, Greenland. Acta Med Scand 1980; 208 : 401-6.
4. Robertson TL, Kato H, Rhoads GG *et al*. Epidemiologic studies of coronary heart disease and stroke in Japanese men living in Japan, Hawaii and California. Am J Carde 1977; 39 : 239-49.
5. Wood DA, Riemersma RA, Butler S *et al*. Linoleic and eicosapentaenoic acids in adipose tissue and platelets and risk of coronary heart disease. Lancet I : 177-183.
6. Bang HO, Dyeberg J. Personal reflections on the Incidence of ischemic heart disease in Oslo during the Second World War. Acta Med Scand 1981; 210 : 245-8.
7. Kromhout D, Bosschieter EB, de Lezenne Coulander C. The inverse relation between fish consumption and 20-year mortality from coronary heart disease. N Engl J Med 1985; 312 : 1205-9.
8. Norell SE, Ahlbom A, Feychting M. Fish consumption and mortality from coronary heart disease, Br Med J 1986; 293 : 426.
9. Shekelle RB, Missell L, Paul O *et al*. Fish consumption and mortality from coronary heart disease. N Engl J Med 1985; 313 : 820.
10. Vollset SE, Heuch I, Bjelke E. Fish consumption and mortality from coronary heart disease. N Engl J Med 1985; 313 : 820-1.
11. Curb JD, Reed DM. Fish consumption and mortality from coronary heart disease. N Engl J Med 1985; 313 : 821.
12. Wahlquist ML, Lo CS, Myers KA. Fish intake and arterial wall characteristics in healthy people and diabetic patients. Lancet II 1989; 944-6.

13. Bang HO, Dyeberg J. Plasma lipids and lipoproteins in Greenlandic west coast Eskimos. Acta Med Scand 1972; 192 : 85-94.

14. Harris WS. Fish oils and plasma lipid and lipoprotein metabolism in humans : a critical review. J Lipid Res 1989; 30 : 785-807.

15. Lorenz R, Spengler U, Fischer S *et al*. Platelet function, thromboxane formation and blood pressure control during supplementation of the western diet with cod liver oil. Circulation 1983; 67 : 504-11.

16. Singer P, Wirth M, Voigt S *et al*. Blood pressure and lipid-lowering effect of mackerel and herring diet in patients with mild essential hypertension. Atherosclerosis 1985; 56 : 223-35.

17. Knapp HR, FitzGerald GA. The antihypertensive effects of fish oil. N Engl J Med 1989; 320 : 1037-43.

18. Friday KE, Childs MT, Tsunehara CH *et al*. Elevated plasma glucose and lowered tri-glyceride levels from Ω-3 fatty acid supplementation in type II diabetes. Diabetes Care 1989; 12 : 276-81.

19. Glauber H, Wallace P, Griver K *et al*. Adverse metabolic effect of Ω-3 fatty acid in non-insulin-dependent diabetes mellitus. Annals Int Med 1988; 108 : 663-8.

20. Schmidt EB, Sorensen PJ, Pedersen JO *et al*. The effect of n-3 polyunsaturated fatty acid on lipids, haemostasis, neutrophil and monocyte chemotaxis in insulin-dependent diabetes mellitus. J Int Med 1989; 225 Suppl 1 : 201-6.

21. Ross R. The pathogenesis of atherosclerosis – an update. N Engl J Med 1986; 314 : 488-500.

22. Dyeberg J, Bang HO, Stoffersen E *et al*. Eicosapentaenoic acid and prevention of thrombosis and atherosclerosis ? Lancet 1978; II : 117-9.

23. Needleman P, Raz A, Minkes MS *et al*. Triene prostaglandins. Prostacyclin and thromboxane biosynthesis and unique biological properties. P Natl Acad Sci USA 1979; 76 : 944-8.

24. Siess W, Roth P, Scherer B *et al*. Platelet membrane fatty acids, platelet aggregation, and thromboxane formation during a mackerel diet. Lancet 1980; I : 441-4.

25. Fischer S, Weber PC. Prostaglandin 13 is formed *in vivo* in man after dietary eicosapentaenoic acid. Nature 1984; 307 : 165-8.

26. V. Schacky C, Weber PC. Metabolism and effects on platelet function of the purified eicosapentaenoic and docosahexaenoic acids in humans. J Clin Invest 1985; 76 : 2446-50.

27. Driss F, Vericel E, Lagarde M *et al*. Inhibition of platelet aggregation and thromboxane synthesis after intake of small amount of eicosapentaenoic acid. Thromb Res 1984; 36 : 389-96.

28. Shimokawa H, Lam JYT, Chesebro JH *et al*. Effects of dietary supplementation with cod liver oil on endothelium-dependent responses in porcine coronary arteries. Circ 1987; 76 : 898-905.

29. Endres S, Ghorbani R, Kelley VE *et al*. The effect of dietary supplementation with n-3 polyunsaturated fatty acids on the synthesis of interleukin-1 and tumor necrosis factor by mononuclear cells. N Engl J Med 1989; 320 : 265-71.

30. Fox PL, DiCorleto PE. Fish oil inhibit endothelial cell production of platelet-derived growth factor-like protein. Science 1988; 241 : 453-6.

31. Barcelli U, Glas-Greenwalt P, Pollak VE. Enhancing effect of dietary supplementation with n-3 fatty acids on plasma fibrinolysis in normal subjects. Thromb Res 1985; 39 : 307-12.

32. Mehta J, Lawson D, Saldeen T. Reduction in plasminogen activator inhibitor-1 with n-3 polyunsaturated fatty acid intake. Am Heart J 1988; 116 : 1201-4.

33. Emeis JJ, van Houvelingen AC, van den Hoogen *et al*. A moderate fish intake increases plasminogen activator inhibitor type-1 in human volunteers. Blood 1989; 74 : 233-37.

34. Leaf A, Weber PC. Cardiovascular effects of n-3 fatty acid. N Engl J Med 1988; 318 : 549-57.

35. Landymore RW, MacAulay M, Sheridan B *et al*. Comparison of cod-liver oil and aspirin-dipyridamole for the prevention of intimal hyperplasia in autologous vein grafts. Ann Thorac Surg 1986; 41 : 54-57.

36. Weiner BH, Ockene IS, Levine PH *et al*. Inhibition of atherosclerosis by cod-liver oil in a hyperlipidemic swine model. N Engl J med 1986; 315 : 841-6.

37. Davis HR, Bridenstein RT, Vesselinovitch D *et al*. Fish oil inhibits development of atherosclerosis in rhesus monkeys. Arteriosclerosis 1987; 7 : 441-9.

38. Thiery J, Seidel D. Fish oil feeding results in an enhancement of cholesterol-induced atherosclerosis in rabbits. Atherosclerosis 1987; 63 : 53-6.

39. Knapp HR, Reilly IAG, Alessandrini P *et al*. *In vivo* indices of platelet and vascular function during fish-oil administration in patients with atherosclerosis. N Engl J Med 1986; 314 : 937-42.

40. Saynor R, Verel D, Gillot T. The long term effect of dietary supplementation with fish lipid concentrate on serum lipids, bleeding time, platelets and angina. Atherosclerosis 1984; 50 : 3-10.

41. Mehta JL, Lopez LM, Lawson D *et al*. Dietary supplementation with n-3 polyunsaturazed fatty acids in patients with stable coronary heart disease. Am J Med 1988; 84 : 45-9.

42. Dehmer GJ, Popma JJ, van den Berg EK *et al*. Reduction in the rate of early restenosis after coronary angioplasty by a diet supplemented with n-3 fatty acids. N Engl J Med 1988; 319 : 733-40.

43. Grigg LE, Kay TW, Valentine PA *et al*. Determinants of restenosis and lack of effect of dietary supplementation with eicosapentaenoic acid on the incidence of coronary artery restenosis after angioplasty. J Am Coll Cardiol 1989; 13 : 665-72.

44. Reis GJ, Boucher TM, Sipperly ME *et al*. Randomised trial of fish oil for prevention of restenosis after coronary angioplasty. Lancet 1989; II : 177-81.

45. Milner MR, Gallino RA, Leffingwell A *et al*. High dose n-3 fatty acid supplementation reduces clinical restenosis after coronary angioplasty. Circ 78; Suppl II-634.

46. Slack JD, Pinkerton CA, Van Tassel J *et al*. Can oral fish oil supplement minimize restenosis after percutaneous transluminal coronary angioplasty ? J Am Coll Card 1987; 9 : 64A.

47. Burr ML, Fehily AM, Gilbert JF *et al*. Effects of changes in fat, fish, and fibre intakes on death and myocardial reinfarction : diet and reinfarction trial (DART). Lancet 1989; II : 757-61.

Fish oil and blood-vessel wall interactions. Eds P.M. Vanhoutte, Ph. Douste-Blazy.
John Libbey Eurotext, Paris © 1991, pp. 141-147.

15

Fatty acids (Ω-3),
Platelets and coronary disease

S. Renaud

INSERM Unit 63, Lyon-Bron, France.

After several decades of discussion it has now been accepted that coronary thrombosis is the preponderant factor leading to myocardial infarction.

The success of thrombosis [1] in re-opening coronary arteries together with the direct observation of thrombi by angioscopy [2] confirm the classical thesis that coronary thrombosis is the cause of myocardial infarction. As far as the thrombus itself is concerned we know that it is formed chiefly by the accumulation of platelets. The crucial role of platelet reactivity in this development has been demonstrated by the rapid effect of small doses of aspirin preventing coronary failure in 50 % of cases of risk syndrome (unstable angina) [4] or even of primary prevention [5]. It has been known for years that aspirin decreases platelet response to aggregation in particular to secondary aggregation induced by ADP [6]. We have moreover recently shown, in collaboration with the Epidemiology Unit of the British Medical Research Council in Cardiff (Wales), in a study of more than 2 000 subjects, that both primary aggregation and secondary ADP induced aggregation increased in myocardial infarction [7]. As a result the prime role of aspirin could be to normalise platelet reactivity; this would explain why aspirin, while it has no effect on lipids, is effective. In fact our studies [7] indicate that platelet reactivity is a major risk factor in myocardial infarction irrespective of the effect of serum lipids (total cholesterol, HDL- cholesterol, triglycerides), of blood pressure or of the use of tobacco.

Nevertheless our previous studies on humans [8-9] and animals [10-11] have shown that the tendency to platelet aggregation depended largely on nutrition, in particular on fat intake. Diet rich in saturated fatty acids increased platelet reactivity. On the other hand, linoleic acid 18 : 2 (Ω-6) the main polyunsaturated fatty acid used to lower cholesterol seems to have a very limited protective effect on platelets.

The only fatty acids likely to lower platelet reactivity would be those of series (Ω-3) whose precursor is alpha-linolenic acid 18 : 3 (Ω-3) found in certain vegetals of the oleaginous variety such as colza and soya. The (Ω-6) and (Ω-3) are the two series of fatty acids indispensable for life which cannot be synthetised in the human organism from simple molecules. The body must therefore absorb the essential precursors, the 18 : 2 (Ω-6) and the 18 : 3 (Ω-3).

The family of the 2 series of essential polyunsaturated fatty acids (Ω-6) and (Ω-3) are :

(Ω-6) 18 : 2 - 18 : 3 - 20 : 3 - 20 : 4 - 22 : 4 - 22 : 5

(Ω-3) 18 : 3 - 18 : 4 - 20 : 4 - 20 : 5 - 22 : 5 - 22 : 6.

3. Fatty acids and platelet reactivity

In an exhaustive survey of the litterature the Dyeberg group concluded that most of the studies on the effect of fish-oils - and hence of 20 : 5 (Ω-3) which they contain in abundance - on ADP and collagen induced platelet aggregation indicated an inhibitory effect [12]. It must nevertheless be emphasised that most of these studies involved a limited number of subjects, over a short period (3-6 weeks) without a control group. The only scientifically satisfactory study involving 60 random volunteers divided into 2 groups, one taking a supplement of 10-16 ml of Ω-3 fatty acid* oil while the control group received the same amount of olive oil, observed no decrease in platelet reactivity, particularly to ADP [13].

It seems likely, as will be seen concerning coronary mortality, that the effect of the Ω-3 and fish oils on platelets depends on the consumption of saturated fats, which would explain the variability of the results in terms of different studies and the subjects'eating habits. The contrasting effects of saturated fats and the Ω-3 on platelets, is clearly demonstrated by the results of our studies on farming populations [9]. From 1976 to 1980, 18 groups of at least 20 farmers per group, were studied in France, Great Britain and

(*) Maxepa®

Belgium. The consumption of saturated fatty acids (SAT) and polyunsaturated 18 : 2, 18 : 3 (Ω-3), 20 : 5 (Ω-3) is displayed in *Figure 1*.

The relationships between platelet aggregation and the fatty acid content of the platelets are shown in *Table I*. It can be seen that in these 18 groups of subjects, there is a significant negative correlation between thrombin, ADP, and collagen induced platelet aggregation and to the fatty acid content of the platelet phospholipids (series Ω-3 ie 20 : 5, 22 : 5 and 22 : 6).

Table I. Analysis of the multiple step by step regression of platelet aggregation related to fatty acid content of platelet phospholipids.

Aggregation	Thrombin	ADP	Collagen
20:3 (Ω-9)	0.44*		0.56*
22:3 (Ω-9)		0.68*	
20:5 (Ω-3)	0.49**		
22:5 (Ω-3)		–0.98**	
22:6 (Ω-3)			–0.61*

*$p < 0.05$; **$p < 0.02$

On the other hand, the platelet reactivity is positively correlated to 20 : 3 or 22 : 3 (Ω-9) platelet content. These fatty acids 20 : 3 and 22 : 3 (Ω-9) are derived from saturated fatty acids 16 : 0 and especially from 18 : 0, the two main saturated fatty acids in the human diet. The higher the consumption of 16 : 0 and 18 : 0 the higher the 20 : 3 and the 22 : 3 (Ω-9) content in the platelets. In our analysis with multiple variants, only these two series of fatty acids furnished the explanation for the platelet reactivity.

Consumption of Ω-3 and coronary disease

The positive role of (Ω-3) fatty acids in reducing platelet reactivity and preventing coronary disease emerged from the studies of Dyerberg and his collaborators among Greenland Eskimos [15]. In spite of a high lipid consumption (almost 40 % of calories) Eskimos hardly suffer from coronary disease. They do, on the other hand, have a tendency to bleed; this led researchers to investigate blood platelets, a primary factor in hemostasis. Nevertheless as illustrated in *Table II* in addition to their high consumption of Ω-3, mainly 20 : 5 (Ω-5) Eskimos consume few saturated fatty acids [16] the environmental factor most closely related to coronary disease [17]. If, generally speaking, fish consumption Economic Cooperation and Develop-

Table II. Comparison between consumption of fats by Eskimos and Danes.

	Eskimos	Danes
Total fats	39	42
Saturated fats	9	22
Ω-3 % Fatty acid	5.3	1.2
Ω-6 % Fatty acid	1.8	4.1
Polyunsaturated/saturated (P/S)	0.84	0.24

Adapted from reference 14

ment Organization (ECDO) countries is compared with the corresponding coronary deaths, it is true that a negative correlation is obtained ($r = 0.38$, $p < 0.05$), which however is too negligeable to be significant [15].

On the other hand, the correlation between the consumption of dairy fats and coronary deaths in the same 21 countries is positive and noticeably higher ($r = 0.78$, $p < 0.001$); this would suggest that the effect of saturated fats in inducing coronary disease is much greater than that of fish in preventing it.

It might be argued that results based on mortality and consumption statistics by country are hardly valid from an epidemiological point of view. However in the case of the particular study of the Seven Countries (Japan, USA, Canada, Italy, France, Great Britain, Germany) whose cohorts were followed up over a period of 15 years, the correlation between the consumption of fish and saturated fats and coronary mortality was the subject of recent studies [19, 20]. The negative correlation between coronary mortality and fish consumption in the 15 cohorts of the study was a somewhat negligeable ($r = 0.26$). On the other hand, the correlation between the consumption of saturated fats and coronary mortality was $r = 0.89$ ($p < 0.001$). These results thus amply confirm the ECDO observations. They suggest that the fatty acids derived from fish cannot be relied upon to offset the harmful effects of an excess of saturated fats. From the point of view of prevention the priority in any modification of eating habits seems to be a reduction in the consumption of saturated fats.

Intervention studies

However, since the consumption of fish is negatively correlated to coronary disease, is it therefore possible to calculate an optimal quantity of fish or Ω-3 with these beneficial effects. In a retrospective study at Zutphen in Holland, Kromhout [21] showed that as little as one fish meal per week gave a degree of protection against coronary disease, this protective effect peaking at 3 meals a week. These results caused surprise at first. But in a recent study, he and his collaborators in Cardiff [22] observed in a dietary study on secondary infarction prevention on 2 000 patients, that neither an increase in linoleic acid nor an increase in cereal fibers, diminished coronary mortality. On the other hand, the consumption of from 1 to 3 fish based meals a week or their equivalent in Ω-3 fatty acid fish oil reduced total mortality by 29 % in 2 years. The greatest decrease (40 %) of mortality through fish was observed in the group consuming the highest quantity of linoleic acid (P/S = 0.8 or more) and in all probability the lowest level of saturated fatty acids.

We have observed in this review article, platelet reactivity, particularly to ADP, in a small number of subjects. The results show that the consumption of 3 fish-based meals a week (about 300 g) almost entirely inhibited secondary ADP-induced aggregation as would aspirin.

It is to be noted that in the fish consuming group a non-significant increase of serum cholesterol was observed.

In a context of secondary prevention of infarction through diet, these results may appear modest. Nevertheless it remains true that the Cardiff study is the first in the field of the secondary prevention of infarction to have reduced total mortality to a significant extent, an effect observed as from the first months of the study. As reviewed recently [23] the major studies of secondary prevention of infarction through changes in eating habits have not reduced significantly total mortality; one of them in fact increased it. Coronary failures were significantly lowered only in the first study. It should be emphasised that in these studies the quantity of polyunsaturated fatty acids in the diet had been inordinately increased (P/S about 1.7 to 2.4).

Conclusions

The demonstration that myocardial infarction is due to coronary thrombosis led to the study of the parameter of hemostasis and more particularly to the reactivity of blood platelets. The striking parallel between known environmental risk factors (saturated fats, alcohol, tobacco...) on coronary disease and on platelet reactivity [9] led research towards factors liable to inhibit this reactivity in order to prevent infarction, the lowering of cholesterol levels alone having frequently been shown to be ineffective, particularly in the short term (less than 3 years) [24].

Aspirin has been the only medecine which until recently, in the course of random testing was able to prevent myocardial infarction efficiently and rapidly. The addition of series Ω-3 fatty acids, particularly those derived from fish oil, seems to have the same rapid effects on platelet reactivity and cardio-vascular morbidity. However the epidemiological studies suggest that a regular high consumption of these Ω-3 fatty acids is not an efficient protection against the harmful effects of saturated fatty acids.

The ideal diet, which remains to be defined, should contain a total of less than 10 % of its calories supplied by saturated fats, together with a substantial consumption of Ω-3 fatty acids. The ratio of series Ω-3 to Ω-6 (linoleic acid) should be approximately 1 to 6 for a P/S situated between 0.5 and 0.7. These measures should also be accompanied by an increased comsumption of cereals, vegetables and fruit, providing the natural anti-oxiders required to stabilise these fatty acids.

References

1. Aims Trial study group. Effect of intravenous APSAC on mortality after acute myocardial infarction : preliminary report of a placebo-controlled clinical trial. Lancet 1988; 1 : 545-9.

2. Forrester JS, Litvack F, Grundfest W *et al.* A perspective of coronary disease seen through the arteries of living man. Circulation 1987; 75 : 505-13.

3. De Wood MA, Spores J, Notske R *et al.* Prevalence of total coronary occlusion during the early hours of transmural myocardial infarction. N Engl J Med 1980; 303 : 897-902.

4. Fuster V, Cohen M, Halpern J. Aspirin in the prevention of coronary disease. N Engl J Med 1989; 321 : 183-5.

5. Steering Committee of the Physician's Health Study Research Group. Final report on the aspirin component of the ongoing Physicians' health study. N Engl J Med 1989; 321 : 129-35.

6. Zucker MB, Peterson J. Inhibition of adenosine diphosphate-induced secondary aggregation and other platelet functions by acetylsalicylic acid ingestion. Proc Soc Exper Biol Med 1968; 127 : 547-51.

7. Elwood PC, Renaud S, Sharp DS *et al.* Ischemic heart disease and platelet aggregation : the Caerphilly collaborative heart disease study (soumis pour publication).

8. Renaud S, Kuba K, Goulet C *et al.* Relationship between platelet fatty acid composition of platelet and platelet aggregation in rat and man. Relation to thrombosis. Circ Res 1970; 26 : 553-64.

9. Renaud S, Morazain R, Godsey F *et al.* Dietary fats, platelet functions and composition in nine groups of French and British farmers. Atherosclerosis 1986; 60 : 37-48.

10. Gautheron P, Renaud S. Hyperlipemia induced hypercoagulable state in rat. Role of an increased activity of platelet phosphatidyl serine in response to certain dietary fatty acids. Thromb Res 1972; 1 : 353-70.

11. McGregor L, Morazain R, Renaud S. A comparison of the effects of dietary short and long chain saturated fatty acids on platelet functions, platelet phospholipids and blood coagulation in rats. Lab Invest 1980; 43 : 438-42.

12. Kristensen SD, Schmidt EB, Dyerberg J. Dietary supplementation with n-3 polyunsaturated fatty acids and human platelet function : a review with particular emphasis on implications for cardiovascular disease. J Intern Med 1989; 225 (Suppl. 1) : 141-150.

13. Rogers S, James KS, Butland BK *et al*. Effects of a fish-oil supplement on serum lipids, rheological variables. Atherosclerosis 1987; 63 : 137-43.

14. Nordoy A, Davenas E, Ciavatti M *et al*. Effect of dietary (n-3) fatty acids on platelet function and lipid metabolism in rats. Biochim Biophys Acta 1985; 835 : 491-500.

15. Dyerberg J, Bang HO, Stoffersen E *et al*. Eicosapentaenoic acid and prevention of thrombosis and atherosclerosis. Lancet 1978; ii : 117-19.

16. Bang HO, Dyerberg J, Sinclair HM. The composition of the Eskimo food in North Western Greenland. Am J Clin Nutr 1980; 33 : 2657-61.

17. Keys A. Coronary heart disease in the Seven Countries. Circulation 1970; 41 (Suppl 1) : 1-211.

18. Crombie IK, McLoone P, Smith WCS *et al*. International differences in coronary heart disease mortality and consumption of fish and other foodstuffs. Eur Heart J 1987; 8 : 560-3.

19. Keys A, Menotti A, Karvonen MJ *et al*. The diet and 15-year death rate in the Seven Countries Study. Am J Epidemiol 1986; 124 : 903-15.

20. Kromhout D. n-3 fatty acids and coronary heart disease : epidemiology from Eskimos to Western populations. J Intern Med 1989, 225 (Suppl. 1) : 47-51.

21. Kromhout D, Bosshieter EB, de Lezenne Coulander C. The inverse relation between fish consumption and 20-year mortality from coronary heart disease. N Engl J Med 1985; 312 : 1205-9.

22. Burr ML, Fehily AM, Gilbert JF *et al*. Effects of changes in fat, fish, and fibre intakes on death and myocardial reinfarction : diet and reinfarction trial (DART). Lancet 1989; 2 : 757-61.

23. Renaud S, de Lorgeril M. Dietary lipids and their relation to ischaemic heart disease : from epidemiology to prevention. J Intern Med 1989; 225 (Suppl. 1): 39-46.

24. Lipid Research Clinics Program. The lipid research clinics coronary primary prevention trial results. JAMA 1984; 251 : 351.

Fish oil and blood-vessel wall interactions. Eds P.M. Vanhoutte, Ph. Douste-Blazy.
John Libbey Eurotext, Paris © 1991, pp. 149-160.

16

Long-term reduction in re-infarction rate, blood fibrinogen, triglyceride and total cholesterol in patients taking Ω-3 fatty acids for ischaemic heart disease

R. Saynor, T. Gillott

Sheffield Cardiothoracic Laboratory, Northern General Hospital, Sheffield, UK.

Abstract

Three hundred and sixty five volunteers suffering from ischaemic heart disease, hyper-lipidaemia or a strong family history of heart attacks had their diets supplemented with Ω-3 fatty acid*, a concentrated fish oil containing 18-19 % eicosapentaenoic acid. No further dietary modification was attempted. We present the first four years of a seven years study.

A significant reduction in serum triglyceride, cholesterol and plasma fibrinogen was observed, together with a significantly increased HDL cholesterol. These beneficial changes persisted to the end of the study. The re-infarction rate in 153 patients who had suffered one or more myocardial infarctions before entering the study were recorded for seven years (918 patient years). Re-infarction was reduced to 1.09 % per year compared to an expected rate in Sheffield of 9 % in with 1980 (the first year of the study) and 4.5 % (the final year of study).

Long term safety was monitored with regard both to clinical chemistry and haemato-logical parameters, none of which was adversely affected by Ω-3 fatty acid consumption.

_____
(*)Maxepa®

R. Saynor, T. Gillott

Introduction

Much attention has focused in recent years on fatty fish and fish oil as a means of improving some coronary heart disease risk factors [1]. A high dietary intake of Ω-3 fatty acids is thought to be responsible for the low incidence of ischaemic heart disease in Eskimos living in the Umanak district of Greenland [2]. A low incidence of ischaemic heart disease has also been reported in coastal-dwelling Turks and Japanese consuming a diet rich in Ω-3 fatty acids [3-6]. Blood lipids in particular appear to be altered by the regular consumption of Ω-3 fatty acids. In 1980, we first reported a significant reduction in serum triglyceride in normal volunteers taking Ω-3 fatty acid* a natural marine triglyceride rich in eicosapentaenoic acid and docosahexaenoic acids [7]. This finding was subsequently confirmed by both open [8-10] and controlled studies in healthy subjects and in patients with ischaemic heart disease [11, 12]. In a further double blind crossover study on hypertriglyceridaemic patients, many of whom had suffered previous myocardial infarcts, we demonstrated a significant superiority of Ω-3 over Ω-6 fatty acids in reducing serum triglyceride and total cholesterol and increasing HDL-C [13].

The bleeding time in Eskimos has been shown to be higher than in the Danes, a group with which the Eskimos have been compared [14, 15]. Other work has demonstrated an increased bleeding time after the consumption of fish oil in British subjects with ischaemic heart disease [16]. Re-occlusion after angioplasty has been shown to be significantly reduced in patients taking Ω-3 fatty acid in addition to aspirin and dipyridamole [17], and indeed many of the reported properties of fish oil would suggest a potential role in the prevention of coronary thrombosis.

This open prospective study was designed to answer two important questions. What are the long-term effects of regular fish oil supplements to the diet on serum triglyceride, total and high density lipoprotein (HDL) cholesterol, fibrinogen and platelet count ? Secondly, does long term supplementation of the diet with fish oil reduce the incidence of myocardial infarction in patients already known to be at high risk ?

(*)Maxepa®

Patients and methods

Three hundred and sixty five subjects participated in the study, of whom 304 were males and 61 were females, with an age range of 18 to 76 years and a median age of 51 years. 47.2 % had suffered a myocardial infarction and 1.9 % had had a stroke prior to joining the study. A total of 49.2 % had a history of angina pectoris, 3.8 % diabetes mellitus and 6.1 % intermittent claudication. Because most of these patients (73 %) had hyperlipidaemia and in view of the pre-existing other high risk factors, it was not considered ethical to give them a placebo, so that this was conducted as an open trial. The study continued over seven years but the data reported here covers the first four years of study. It was considered, with the exception of re-infarction rates, that insufficient numbers of subjects had completeled the full seven yeras for full statistical analysis.

Seventy five patients withdrew from the study over seven years. The commonest reasons for withdrawal were moving away from the area and dislike of the taste of the fish oil which was taken by spoonful since capsules had not yet been devised. On joining the study, 199 patients were receiving medication for cardiovascular disorders, including treatment for angina and hypertension. Nine had been taking clofibrate but discontinued this before joining the study. No patient taking aspirin was included in the study.

Ω-3 fatty acid, a selected whole body fish oil containing 18-19 % eicosapentaenoic acid (EPA), was kindly supplied by Seven Seas Health Care Ltd, Hull, UK. Serum for lipid and routine biochemical estimations was separated from venous blood withdrawn with minimum stasis after a 12-14 hour fast. Blood for haematological estimations was collected into EDTA. Two blood samples for lipid measurement were taken at seven days intervals before supplementation of the diet with Ω-3 fatty acid and further samples were taken at 1, 3, 6, 12, 18, 24, 30, 36, 42, and 48 months after starting Ω-3 fatty acid. In order to avoid diurnal lipid changes, all blood samples were taken between 9.00 and 10.00 a.m. During the first year of study, each participant was asked to take 10 ml Ω-3 fatty acid (1.8 g EPA) twice daily with food. No further modification of the diet was attempted and, to try to avoid the complicating effects of concomitant other dietary manipulations, patients were encouraged to stay on the same diet as when they first joined the study. Subsequently the dose was reduced to 10 ml once daily.

Laboratory assays

Serum triglyceride, total cholesterol and high density lipoprotein cholesterol (HDL-C) were measured as previously described [16]. Bleeding times were

151

measured by the modified «Simplate» method and platelets were counted on a Coulter counter. To prospectively assess the long term safety of Ω-3 fatty acid, routine haematological and clinical chemistry profiles were measured by the respective laboratories of this hospital using the Technicon H6000 and Vickers SP120 instruments. Plasma fibrinogen was measured by the Coagulation Laboratory [18].

Statistics

A method based on piecewise linear interpolation [19], carried out for each individual patient, was used on each of the following variables : serum triglyceride, total cholesterol, HDL-C, plasma fibrinogen and platelet count.

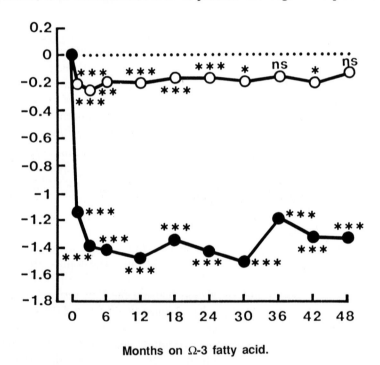

Months on Ω-3 fatty acid.

Figure 1. Total serum triglyceride levels (mmol/l), mean change from baseline.
.... No change
—o— Baseline 1.97 mmol/l
—●— Baseline 1.97 mmol/l
*** Significant at 0.1 % level
 **   Significant at 1 % level
  *   Significant at 5 % level

Results

Serum triglyceride levels in the group of subjects with raised baseline levels (mean 3.76 mmol/l) fell significantly within one month as did the triglyceride levels in the group with «normal» baseline levels (mean 1.35 mmol/l). In both groups the changes were significant at the 0.1 % level. Normal levels were defined as <1.97 mmol/l. These results are shown in *Figure 1*.

Serum cholesterol in the group of subjects with raised baseline levels (mean 8.15 mmol/l) was reduced at one month (significant at 0.1 % level). The group with a baseline <6.5 mmol/l (mean 5.64 mmol/l) showed no significant change throughout the study *(Figure 2)*.

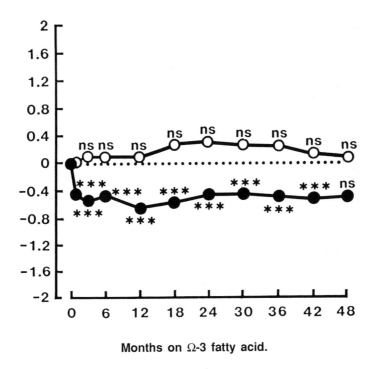

Months on Ω-3 fatty acid.

Figure 2. Total serum cholesterol levels (mmol/l), Mean change from baseline.
.... No change
—o— Baseline 6.5 mmol/l
—•— Baseline 6.5 mmol/l
*** Significant at 0.1 % level
** Significant at 1 % level
* Significant at 5 % level

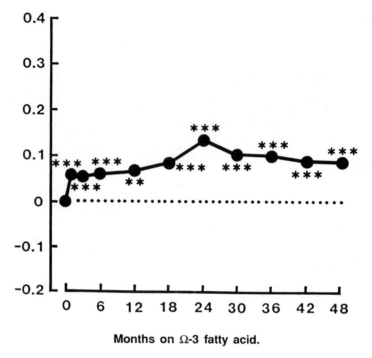

Figure 3. Serum HDL cholesterol levels (mmol/l) mean change from baseline.
.... No change
—●— All patients
*** Significant at 0.1 % level
** Significant at 1 % level

At each timepoint mean HDL cholesterol levels showed an increase from baseline levels (mean 1.22 mmol/l). These increases are shown in *Figure 3*. Furthermore, at each timepoint a majority of patients were found to have increased levels significant at 0.1 % level for each timepoint).

Plasma fibrinogen levels demonstrated mean reductions from baseline levels at each timepoint and these tended to increase in magnitude as time progressed *(Figure 4)*. After one month, the mean fibrinogen level was reduced by 0.14 g/l, at six months the observed mean reduction from baseline levels was 0.33 g/l and at 48 months the mean reduction was 0.89 g/l (significant at the 0.1 % level). No significant change in mean platelet count was observed during this study.

Of the 153 patients included in this study who had had one or more myocardial infarctions before inclusion, seven had one additional myocardial infarction and one had two additional myocardial infarctions during the seven

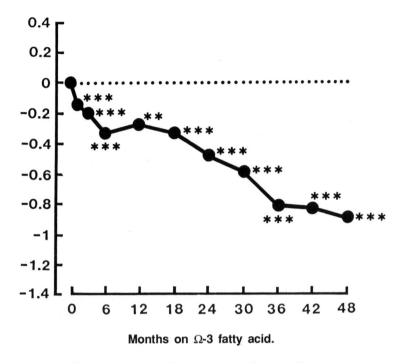

Figure 4. Plasma fibrinogen levels (g/l), mean change from baseline.
.... No change
——●—— All patients
  *** Significant at 0.1 % level
   ** Significant at 1 % level

years of taking Ω-3 fatty acid. Four of these patients died. An additional patient, who was excluded from the statistics, died of a myocardial infarction five months after he had discontinued Ω-3 fatty acid, this patient having taken the fish oil for only a single month. These 153 post-infarction patients who were included in the study contributed a total of 918 patient years, and suffered an annual re-infarction rate of 1.09 % *(Figure 5)*. Four further patients died while taking part in the study, two as a result of road traffic accidents, one from emphysema - the cause of death in the fourth, who dropped out from the trial having left the area, is unknown to us. In 1980 the annual re-infarction rate in the Sheffield district was 9 % and in 1987 it was 4.5 % per annum [20].

A further 58 patients had angina when they began the study and 56 others had no symptoms but a strong family history of heart disease. None of either group suffered a myocardial infarction during the seven years of the study.

155

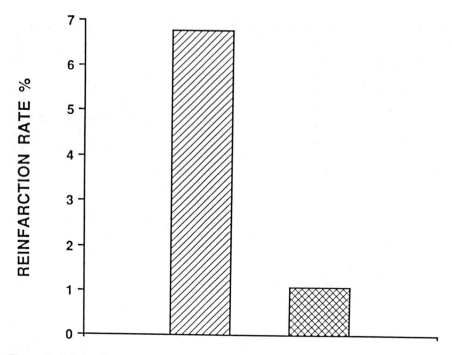

Figure 5. Reinfarction rate.
▨▨▨ Mean reinfarction rate on conventional treatment (1980-87).
▩▩▩ Mean reinfarction rate on conventional treatment plus Ω-3 fatty acid (1980-87).

Ω-3 fatty acid was found to be without side-effect over this long period of medication. Although up to 17.5 % of patients had minor disturbances of one or more of the routine chemical and haematological parameters, these changes were small and inconsistent and were felt to be of no significance. No change in any parameter could be attributed to Ω-3 fatty acid.

Discussion

A recent editorial sounded a cautionary note on both the safety and the long-term efficacy of fish oil in lowering plasma triglyceride [21]. Anxiety had been raised by two published studies. In the first study a different fish oil concentrate (Ω-500, Omegacaps, Missouri 15 g daily had failed to sustain the initial reduction of plasma triglycerides in 16 patients over six months of study [22]. In the second study three cans of mackerel a week failed to sustain an initial lowering of triglyceride in 12 patients over eight months [23]. Our much longer study in much larger numbers of patients found Ω-3 fatty acid to be both safe and to show a persistent reduction in triglyceride concentrations, which was as effective after four years as during the initial period of study. While the dose of oil given in the mackerel study was small and therefore suggests a possible explanation for the loss of long term efficacy, we cannot explain the reduction in long term efficacy in the Ω-500 trial, where the maintenance dose of Ω-3 fatty acid was 3.9 g/day. Other studies have however tended to confirm our findings [24-26]. One possible explanation for these differences might lie in the different composition of fish oils produced by different manufacturers.

The mechanism by which fish oil reduces plasma triglyceride has been discussed at length elsewhere [16, 27-29]. Hypertriglyceridaemia is a univariate risk factor for ischaemic heart disease but its role as an independent risk factor is still controversial. However, a strong relationship between non-fasting VLDL levels and cardiovascular mortality in both men and women has been reported [30]. This suggests that triglyceride rich lipoprotein in random samples is an important predictor of both total and cardiovascular mortality. Hypertriglyceridaemia has also been associated with depressed fibrinolysis, an important factor in ischaemic heart disease [31]. An association between hypertriglyceridaemia and increased plasma concentrations of fibrinogen has been reported to be partially corrected by reducing the plasma triglycerides [32].

Most myocardial infarctus are the result of thrombotic occlusion. A number of prospective studies have shown plasma fibrinogen to be a highly significant risk factor in the development of coronary heart disease [33-37]. In one of these studies [37] platelet aggregability was strongly associated with plasma fibrinogen concentration. A strong correlation has been reported between a decreased red cell filterability, high triglyceride, high fibrinogen and low HDL-C levels. The present work suggests a positive correlation between triglyceride and fibrinogen. Reducing triglyceride and maintening a low plasma level may result in a lessening of its adverse effects on haemorrheology and damage to the arterial wall. The foregoing would appear to suggest a link wither directly or indirectly between serum triglyceride, plasma fibrinogen and platelet aggregation which would not only lead to a hypercoagulable state but might also stimulate atherogenesis. It is suggested that the pathological processes leading to thrombotic occlusion may be beneficially modified by increasing the level of Ω-3 series fatty acids in the circulating blood.

The fall of 11 % in total serum cholesterol over four years in patients with raised baseline levels was consistent and significant. Increases in HDL cholesterol were highly significant at each time point and may be related to the fall in serum triglycerides. The increased HDL-C is suggestive of an enhanced removal of cholesterol and that a shift in body cholesterol from the serum to the tissue pool is not the mechanism by which the total cholesterol is reduced. The ingestion of Ω-3 fatty acids appears to lead to a reduction in triglyceride-rich VLDL and consequently it appears likely that the synthesis and release of apo A-I from endothelial cells is increased. This probably leads to increased conversion of discoid to spherical HDL due to the activating effect of the apoprotein on lecithin cholesterol acyl transferase (LCAT). It is also possible that an increase in HDL synthesis occurs by stimulation of the end process of HDL formation, allowing for a greater rate of apo A-I incorporation into the final HDL.

Although changes in platelet count did not reach significance, about 50 % of subjects experienced a reduction in platelet numbers. The incorporation of Ω-3 fatty acids into the platelet membrane lipids leads to the partial replacement of arachidonic acid in the membrane by eicosapentaenoic acid, which in turn leads to the weak aggregating agent, thromboxane A3, instead of the potent aggregator A2 [37], thereby reducing the tendency to thrombosis.

It has been shown in an intermediate term study of two years duration that the consumption of fatty fish or as little as 3 ml daily of Ω-3 fatty acid resulted in a 30 % reduction of re-infarction when compared with patients who did not increase their fish oil consumption [38]. The reduction in re-infarction rate in our study was more than 70 % in spite of the fact that the study extended over 7 years. It is possible that the more dramatic reduction in re-infarction rate in our subjects was due to the larger doses of fish oil consumed (10 ml daily). Our results are encouraging and point to the need for large population studies for confirmation. However some caution may be necessary in evaluating the results of studies which involve different formulations of Ω-3 fatty acids since these may not give identical results.

Acknowledgments

We wish to thank Dr D. Verel, former Consultant Cardiologist and Dr GDG. Oakley, Consultant Cardiologist for permission to study their patients. Thanks are due to the staff of the Cardiothoracic Laboratory for their continuing help and to Mr D. Chalmers and Miss S. Allen for their invaluable assistance with the statistics. We are most grateful to Seven Seas Health Care Ltd. for providing generous supplies of Ω-3 fatty acid from 1980 to 1987. Finally, we are indebted to Dr F.P. Ryan for constructive criticism of the draft.

References

1. Herold PM, Kinsella JE. Fish Oil consumption and decreased risk of cardiovascular disease : a comparison of findings from animal and human trials. Am J Clin Nutr 1986; 43 : 566-570.

2. Bang HO, Dyeberg J, Hjorne N. The composition of food-consumed by Greenland Eskimos. Acta Med Scand 1976; 200 : 69-71.

3. Yotakis LDO. The preventive effect of the polyunsaturated fats and trombosis. Thromb Haemostas 1981; 46 : 65 abstr.

3. Kato H, Tillotson J, Nichamal MZ *et al*. Epidemiological studies of coronary heart disease and stroke in Japanese men living in Japan, Hawaii and California : serum lipids and diet. Am J Epidemiol 1975; 102 : 372-385.

5. Worth RM, Kato H, Rhoads GG *et al*. Epidemiological studies of coronary heart disease and stroke in Japanese men living in Japan, Hawaii and California : mortality. Am J Epidemiol 1975; 102 : 481-490.

6. Hirai A, Hamazaki T, Terano T *et al*. Eicosapentaenoic acid and platelet function in Japanese. Lancet 1980; ii : 1132-33.

7. Saynor R, Verel D. Effect of a marine oil high in eicosapentaenoic acid on blood lipids and coagulation. IRCS Med Sci 1980; 8 : 378-9.

8. Saynor R, Verel D, Gillott T. EPA, bleeding time, platelets, serum lipids and GTN consumption. Proc VI Int Thromb Haemostas, (Stockholm) 1983; 50 (1) : 136 abstr.

9. Sanders TAB, Roshanai F. The influence of different types of Ω-3 polyunsaturated fatty acids on blood lipids and platelet function in healthy volunteers. Clin Sci 1983; 64 : 91-99.

10. Harris WS, Connor WE, Inkeless SB *et al*. Dietary Ω-3 fatty acid prevent carbohydrate-induced hypertriglyceridaemia. Metabolism 1984; 33 : 1016-19.

11. Dyerberg J, Bang HO. A hypothesis on the development of acute myocardial infarction in Greenlanders. Scan J Clin Lab Invest 1982; 42 : 7-13.

12. Nestel PJ, Connor WE, Reardon MF *et al*. Suppression by diets rich in fish oil of very low density lipoprotein in man. J Clin Invest 1984; 74 : 82-89.

13. Saynor R, Gillott T, Doyle T *et al*. Clinical studies on the effect of dietary, n-3 and n-6 fatty acids on serum lipids, haemostasis and GTN consumption. Prog Lipid Res 1986; 25 : 211-217.

14. Dyeberg J, Bang HO. Lipid metabolism, atherogenesis and haemostasis in Eskimos : the role of the prostaglandin-3 family. Haemostasis 1979; 8 : 227-233.

15. Sinclair HM. Prevention of coronary heart disease : the role of essential fatty acids. Postgrad Med J 1980; 56 : 579-584.

16. Saynor R, Verel D, Gillott T. The long-term effect of dietary supplementation with fish lipid concentrate on serum lipids, bleeding time, platelets and angina. Atherosclerosis 1984; 50 : 3-10.

17. Dehmer GJ, Popma JJ, van den Berg EK *et al*. Reduction in the rate of early restenosis after coronary angioplasty by a diet supplemented with n-3 fatty acids. New Engl J Med 1988; 319 (12) : 734-739.

18. Burmester HBC, Aulton K, Horsfield GI. Evaluation of a rapid method for the determination of plasma fibrinogen. J Clin Path 1970; 23 : 43-46.

19. Gans DJ. A simple method based on broken lines interpolation for displaying data from long-term clinical trials. Statistics in Medicine 1982; 1 : 131-137.

20. Verel D. Personal communication.

21. Editorial. Fish oil revisited. Lancet 1989; ii : 427-428.

22. Schectman G, Kaul S, Cherayil GD *et al*. Can the hypotriglyceridemic effect of fish oil concentrate be sustained ? Ann Intern Med 1989; 110 : 346-352.

23. Singer P, Berger I, Luck K *et al*. Long term effect of mackerel diet on blood pressure, serum lipids and thromboxane formation in patients with mild essential hypertension. Atherosclerosis 1986; 62 : 259-265.

24. Hamazaki T, Nakazawa JR, Tateno S *et al*. Effects of fish oil rich in eicosapentaenoic acid on serum lipid in hyperlipidemic haemodialysis patients. Kidney Int 1984; 26 : 81-84.

25. Simons LA, Hickie JB, Balasubramanian S. On the effects of dietary n-3 fatty acid (Maxepa®) on plasma lipids and lipoproteins in patients with hyperlipidemia. Atherosclerosis 1985; 54 : 75-88.

26. Miller JP, Heath ID, Choraria SK *et al*. Triglyceride lowering effect of MaxEPA® fish lipid concentrate : a multicentre placebo controlled double blind study. Clinica Chemica Acta 1988; 251-260.

27. Iritani N, Inoguchi K, Endo M *et al*. Identification of shellfish fatty acids and their effects on lipogenic enzymes. Biochem Biophys 1980; 618 : 378-382.

28. Yang Y-T, Williams MA. Comparison of C18, C20 and C22 unsaturated fatty acids in reducing fatty acid synthesis in isolated rat hepatocytes. Biophys Acta 1978; 531 : 133-150.

29. Saynor R. The effects of diatery n-3 fatty acid on serum lipids and haemostasis in man. Ph D Thesis 1984 University of Sheffield.

30. Anderson KM, Kannel WB, Wilson PWF *et al*. Non-fasting VLDL and long-term cardiovascular mortality : The Framington Study. In preparation.

31. Glas-Greenwalt P, Kashyap ML, Ahmad M *et al*. Hypertriglyceridaemia is associated with depressed fibrinolysis. Blood 1984; 64 : 256a.

32. Mikhailidis DP, Barradas MA, Dandona P. Cardiovascular risk in patients with treated familial hypertriglyceridaemia. J R Soc Med 1987; 80 : 61-63.

33. Wilhelmsen L, Svardsudd K, Korsan-Bengtsen K *et al*. Fibrinogen as a risk factor for stroke and myocardial infarction. New Engl J Med 1984; 311 : 501-505.

34. Stone MC, Thorpe JM. Plasma fibrinogen - a major coronary risk factor. J R Coll Gen Pract 1985; 35 : 565-569.

35. Meade TW, Brozovic M, Chakrabarti RR. Haemostatic function and ischaemic heart disease : principal results of the Northwick Park Heart Study. Lancet 1986; ii : 533-537.

36. Kannel WB, D'Agostino RB, Belanger AJ. Fibrinogen cigarette smoking and the risk of cardiovascular disease : Insights from the Framingham Study. Amer Heart J 1987; 113 : 1006-1010.

37. Needleman P, Whittaker MO, Wyche A *et al*. Manipulation of platelet aggregation by prostaglandins and their fatty acid precursors : Pharmacological basis for a therapeutic approach. Prostaglandins 1980; 19 : 165-171.

38. Burr ML, Fehily AM, Gilbert JF *et al*. Effects of changes in fat, fish and fibre intakes on death and myocardial re-infarction diet and re-infarction trial (DART). Lancet 1989; ii : 757-761.

Fish oil and blood-vessel wall interactions. Eds P.M. Vanhoutte, Ph. Douste-Blazy.
John Libbey Eurotext, Paris © 1991, pp. 161-162.

17

Prevention of restenosis
after transluminal angioplasty
(Preliminary report)

Schmitz and Dehmer conducted a study designed to assess the advantages
and the harmlessness of Ω-3 fatty acid treatment in the prevention of precocious restenoses after coronary angioplasty.

The epidemiological data would suggest that in fact the addition to the diet
of fish oils rich in unsaturated Ω-3 fatty acids does have a protective effect
against atherosclerosis.

This random double blind test compared one group treated with Ω-3 fatty
acid* with another undergoing treatment by aspirin and dipyridamole. The
protective effect of Ω-3 fatty acid was tested on 103 coronary lesions, or
83 high-risk male subjects.

In this type of assessment the first difficulty is to determine how the restenoses should be measured : the measurement technique employed must be
sufficiently reliable to permit definite conclusions.

The work of Schmitz and Dehmer upholds the argument of a beneficial
effect from Ω-3 fatty acid in terms of restenosis prevention, taking into account the assessment methods used by the authors. Other wider studies will
nevertheless be required to confirm these results.

---

*Maxepa®.

Some studies are yet more convincing, but here again the methods used should be born in mind before reaching a final judgement.

After a follow-up of six months, 22 patients were re-examined for recurrent symptoms. Angiographically demonstrated restenoses appeared in 13 patients (18 %). Moreover 45 patients subjected to angioplasty during the same period received Ω-3 unsaturated fatty acids before or after the operation; we could thus see that restenosis was less frequent in patients treated with Ω-3 fatty acid.

Author Index